high protein cookbook

FOR WEIGHT LOSS

mark primitive

ZERO-STRESS

Copyright © 2025 by Mark Primitive

All rights reserved.

No part of this book may be reproduced in any form or by any electronic or mechanical means, including information storage and retrieval systems, without written permission from the author, except for the use of brief quotations in a book review.

contents

Introduction	vii
1. BREAKFAST RECIPES	**1**
Protein-Packed Omelette	1
Greek Yogurt Parfait	2
Spinach and Egg Muffins	2
High Protein Pancakes	3
Breakfast Burrito	3
Cottage Cheese and Fruit Bowl	4
Avocado and Egg Toast	4
Chia Seed Protein Pudding	5
Smoked Salmon Bagel	5
Almond Butter Banana Toast	6
Breakfast Egg and Veggie Skillet	6
Berry Smoothie Bowl	7
Turkey Sausage and Egg Muffins	7
Overnight Protein Oats	8
Scrambled Egg Whites with Veggies	8
Banana Nut Protein Bread	9
Quinoa Breakfast Bowl	9
Egg and Cheese Wrap	10
Tofu Scramble	10
Protein French Toast	11
2. LUNCH RECIPES	**12**
Grilled Chicken Salad	12
Tuna Avocado Wrap	13
Quinoa and Chickpea Bowl	13
High Protein Cobb Salad	14
Turkey and Veggie Sandwich	14
Lentil Soup	15
Chicken Caesar Wrap	15
Greek Salad with Grilled Chicken	16
Egg Salad Lettuce Wraps	16
Salmon Sushi Bowl	17
Black Bean Burrito Bowl	17
Chicken Fajita Salad	18
Protein Pasta Primavera	18
Shrimp and Quinoa Salad	19
Avocado Chicken Wrap	19
High Protein Chili	20
Mediterranean Chicken Bowl	20
Asian Tofu Salad	21
Turkey Burger Lettuce Wrap	21
Lentil and Veggie Stir-fry	22

Salmon Avocado Salad	22
Chickpea Protein Wrap	23
Spinach & Turkey Meatballs	23
Spicy Tuna Salad Bowl	24
Veggie Omelette Wrap	24
High Protein Buddha Bowl	25
Egg and Tuna Salad	25
Grilled Chicken and Veggie Wrap	26
Steak Salad with Protein Dressing	26
Protein-Packed Turkey Soup	27
3. DINNER RECIPES	**28**
Garlic Herb Grilled Salmon	28
Chicken and Broccoli Stir-fry	29
Protein-Rich Turkey Meatloaf	29
Steak with Grilled Vegetables	30
Oven-Baked Cod with Herbs	30
Chicken Quinoa Bowl	31
Baked Stuffed Bell Peppers	31
High-Protein Beef Stir-fry	32
Salmon and Asparagus Foil Pack	32
Shrimp and Vegetable Skewers	33
Turkey and Sweet Potato Skillet	33
Grilled Chicken with Avocado Salsa	34
Zucchini Noodles with Turkey Meatballs	34
Spicy Chicken & Veggie Bowl	35
Grilled Tuna Steaks	35
Herb Roasted Chicken Breast	36
Beef and Broccoli Protein Bowl	36
Chicken Cauliflower Fried Rice	37
Baked Tilapia with Veggies	37
High-Protein Taco Salad	38
Spaghetti Squash with Turkey Bolognese	38
Chicken Parmesan (Low-Carb)	39
Spicy Shrimp Stir-fry	39
Italian Meatball Bake	40
Grilled Pork Chops with Veggies	40
Teriyaki Chicken Protein Bowl	41
Lemon Garlic Chicken Breasts	41
Turkey Zucchini Burgers	42
Baked Salmon with Dill Sauce	42
Protein Veggie Lasagna	43
4. MAIN VEGETARIAN RECIPES	**44**
Chickpea & Quinoa Salad	44
Tofu & Veggie Stir-fry	45
High-Protein Lentil Curry	45
Black Bean Veggie Burger	46
Crispy Tofu & Edamame Stir-Fry	46
Spicy Bean Chili	47

Protein Pasta with Spinach and Chickpeas	47
Vegan Buddha Bowl	48
Mushroom & Lentil Tacos	48
High Protein Falafel Wrap	49
Chickpea Salad Sandwich	49
Black Bean Enchiladas	50
Vegetarian Eggplant Parmesan	50
Quinoa and Veggie Protein Bowl	51
Lentil and Mushroom Burgers	51
5. SIDES RECIPES	**52**
Roasted Garlic Broccoli	52
Quinoa Salad	53
Cauliflower Rice	53
Grilled Asparagus with Lemon	54
Edamame & Veggie Salad	54
Roasted Brussels Sprouts	55
High Protein Bean Salad	55
Garlic Roasted Green Beans	56
Cucumber & Chickpea Salad	56
Baked Sweet Potato Fries	57
Creamy Spinach & Greek Yogurt	57
Veggie & Lentil Medley	58
Roasted Veggie Mix	58
Tomato and Basil Quinoa	59
Protein-Rich Coleslaw	59
6. SNACK RECIPES	**60**
Protein Energy Balls	60
Greek Yogurt & Berry Bowl	61
Cottage Cheese & Pineapple	61
Peanut Butter Protein Bars	62
Tuna & Cucumber Bites	62
Protein-Packed Trail Mix	63
Avocado Egg Salad Bites	63
Protein Yogurt Smoothie	64
Roasted Chickpeas	64
Almond Butter & Apple Slices	65
Turkey & Cheese Roll-ups	65
Protein Veggie Muffins	66
Edamame Snack Bowl	66
Egg Salad Celery Boats	67
Protein Chocolate Shake	67
7. DESSERT RECIPES	**68**
Protein Chocolate Mousse	68
Greek Yogurt Cheesecake Cups	69
High Protein Banana Bread	69
Chocolate Avocado Protein Brownies	70
Vanilla Protein Pudding	70

Peanut Butter Protein Cookies — 71
Protein Fruit Crumble — 71
Protein Ice Cream — 72
Chia Seed Protein Cookies — 72
Protein Cheesecake Bites — 73
Chocolate Protein Pancake Stack — 73
Strawberry Protein Sorbet — 74
Protein Lemon Bars — 74
Banana Chocolate Chip Protein Muffins — 75
Coconut Protein Truffles — 75

8. 60 DAY MEAL PLAN — 76

Acknowledgments — 81

introduction

Welcome to the High Protein Cookbook for Weight Loss!

If you're looking for a way to transform your health, achieve your ideal weight, and boost your daily energy, you've come to the right place. This cookbook is your essential guide to making high-protein meals a delicious and sustainable part of your lifestyle. Whether you're aiming to **lose weight, build lean muscle, or simply adopt healthier eating habits**, a diet rich in protein is one of the most effective ways to support your goals.

why focus on high-protein meals?

Protein is one of the most important macronutrients when it comes to weight loss and overall health. Unlike carbohydrates and fats, protein takes longer to digest, helping you stay full for extended periods. This means **fewer cravings, less snacking, and better appetite control**. Additionally, protein plays a crucial role in preserving muscle mass while burning fat, keeping your metabolism active and promoting a leaner physique.

the basics of a high protein diet for weight loss

A high-protein diet focuses on **lean protein sources** such as chicken, fish, eggs, legumes, dairy, and plant-based proteins. Incorporating these foods into your meals provides several benefits:

✅ **Increased Satiety** – Helps reduce hunger and prevent overeating.

✅ **Muscle Preservation** – Supports lean muscle while losing fat.

✅ **Higher Metabolic Rate** – Burns more calories during digestion.

✅ **Steady Energy Levels** – Prevents energy crashes associated with carb-heavy meals.

essential ingredients for your pantry

A well-stocked pantry makes it easier to prepare high-protein meals effortlessly. Here are the must-have ingredients to keep on hand:

- **Lean Protein Sources:** Canned tuna, chicken breast, turkey, lean beef jerky.
- **Plant-Based Proteins:** Lentils, beans, chickpeas, quinoa, nuts, seeds.

- **Healthy Fats:** Olive oil, avocado oil, coconut oil, nut butters.
- **Whole Grains & Fiber:** Brown rice, oats, whole-grain pasta, chia seeds, flaxseeds.
- **Flavor Enhancers:** Herbs, spices, low-sodium broths, vinegars, lemon juice.

cooking tips and techniques

Preparing high-protein meals doesn't have to be time-consuming or difficult. With these simple cooking techniques, you can enjoy **delicious, nutrient-rich meals** without the hassle:

🔍 **Batch Cooking:** Grill chicken, roast vegetables, or cook lentils in advance to save time.

🔥 **Efficient Cooking Methods:** Grilling, baking, steaming, and air frying help retain nutrients without extra calories.

🔪 **Proper Portioning:** Avoid overeating by measuring portions accurately.

🌿 **Flavor Without Calories:** Use fresh herbs, spices, and citrus juices instead of heavy sauces.

how to plan and prep meals efficiently

Meal planning is key to **sticking to your nutrition goals** and avoiding unhealthy last-minute choices. Follow these steps to stay organized:

📌 **Plan Your Week** – Select recipes in advance and create a shopping list.

🥗 **Prep Ahead** – Chop vegetables, marinate proteins, and portion snacks to save time.

🍱 **Smart Storage** – Use airtight containers for easy meal access throughout the week.

🔄 **Stay Flexible** – Adjust recipes based on your schedule and cravings to maintain variety.

With these **practical tips and high-protein meal ideas**, you're now ready to embark on your journey toward a healthier, more energetic lifestyle—one delicious meal at a time. Let's get started! 🚀🍽️

breakfast recipes

...

Kickstart Your Day the Right Way

Breakfast sets the tone for your day, and starting with a high-protein meal helps control hunger, stabilize blood sugar, and enhance mental clarity. These easy, nutritious recipes will energize you and keep you satisfied until lunchtime.

protein-packed omelette

Ingredients (2 servings):

- 4 large eggs
- ½ cup spinach, chopped
- ¼ cup diced bell peppers
- ¼ cup diced onions
- ½ cup shredded cheddar cheese
- Salt and pepper to taste
- 1 tablespoon olive oil

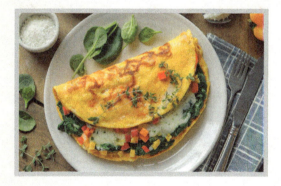

Instructions:

Whisk eggs in a bowl and season with salt and pepper. - Heat olive oil in a skillet over medium heat. - Add onions and bell peppers, cook for 2 minutes until soft. - Pour eggs into skillet, cook until nearly set, then sprinkle spinach and cheese over half of the omelette. - Fold the omelette over the filling and cook for an additional 1-2 minutes. - Serve immediately.

Nutritional Information (per serving):

Calories: 310 | Protein: 21g | Carbohydrates: 6g | Dietary Fiber: 1g | Sugars: 3g | Fat: 23g (Total), 8g (Saturated) | Cholesterol: 370mg | Sodium: 380mg

greek yogurt parfait

Ingredients (2 servings):
- 1½ cups plain Greek yogurt (low-fat or non-fat)
- 1 cup mixed berries (strawberries, blueberries, raspberries)
- ¼ cup low-sugar granola
- 1 tablespoon raw honey (optional)

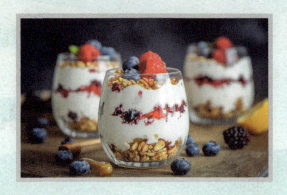

Instructions:

Layer Greek yogurt evenly into two clear glasses or bowls. - Add mixed berries over yogurt, then sprinkle granola on top. - Repeat layers until all ingredients are used. - Drizzle honey on top, if desired. - Serve immediately or refrigerate briefly.

Nutritional Information (per serving):

Calories: 240 | Protein: 18g | Carbohydrates: 26g | Dietary Fiber: 3g | Sugars: 15g | Fat: 7g (Total), 2g (Saturated) | Cholesterol: 10mg | Sodium: 60mg

---

spinach and egg muffins

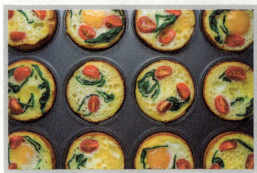

Ingredients (2 servings):
- 4 large eggs
- ½ cup fresh spinach, chopped
- ¼ cup cherry tomatoes, diced
- ¼ cup grated parmesan cheese
- Salt and pepper to taste
- Cooking spray (oil-based)

Instructions:

Preheat oven to 375°F (190°C). - Spray a muffin tin with cooking spray. - Whisk eggs in a bowl and season with salt and pepper. - Mix spinach, cherry tomatoes, and parmesan into the eggs. - Divide evenly among 4 muffin cups. - Bake for 18-20 minutes, until golden and firm. - Allow to cool slightly before removing from tin.

Nutritional Information (per serving - 2 muffins):

Calories: 220 | Protein: 17g | Carbohydrates: 4g | Dietary Fiber: 1g | Sugars: 2g | Fat: 15g (Total), 6g (Saturated) | Cholesterol: 370mg | Sodium: 340mg

high protein pancakes

Ingredients (2 servings):
- ½ cup oatmeal
- ½ cup low-fat cottage cheese
- 2 large eggs
- ½ teaspoon vanilla extract
- ¼ teaspoon cinnamon
- Cooking spray
- ½ cup fresh berries (optional topping)

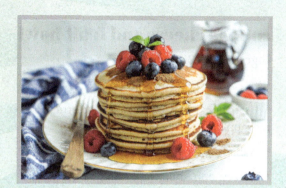

Instructions:

Combine oatmeal, cottage cheese, eggs, vanilla, and cinnamon in a blender; blend until smooth. - Heat a non-stick skillet over medium heat and spray lightly with cooking spray. - Pour batter to form small pancakes, cooking until bubbles form. - Flip pancakes and cook another 2 minutes until golden. - Serve warm, topped with fresh berries if desired.

Nutritional Information (per serving):

Calories: 280 | Protein: 20g | Carbohydrates: 24g | Dietary Fiber: 3g | Sugars: 4g | Fat: 11g (Total), 3g (Saturated) | Cholesterol: 190mg | Sodium: 300mg

---

breakfast burrito

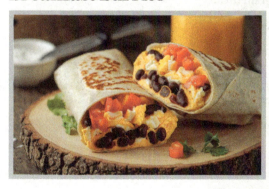

Ingredients (2 servings):
- 4 large eggs
- ½ cup black beans, rinsed and drained
- ¼ cup diced tomatoes
- ¼ cup diced onions
- ½ cup shredded low-fat cheddar cheese
- 2 whole-wheat tortillas (medium size) -
- Salt and pepper to taste - 1 tablespoon olive oil

Instructions:

Whisk eggs with salt and pepper in a bowl. - Heat olive oil in a skillet over medium heat. - Add onions and tomatoes, sauté for 2 minutes. - Add eggs, scramble gently until almost set, then stir in black beans. - Divide egg mixture between tortillas, sprinkle cheese on top, and fold into burritos. - Serve warm.

Nutritional Information (per serving - 1 burrito):

Calories: 340 | Protein: 22g | Carbohydrates: 29g | Dietary Fiber: 6g | Sugars: 3g | Fat: 16g (Total), 5g (Saturated) | Cholesterol: 380mg | Sodium: 410mg

cottage cheese and fruit bowl

Ingredients (2 servings):

- 1½ cups low-fat cottage cheese
- 1 cup fresh mixed fruits (strawberries, blueberries, peaches, pineapple)
- 2 tablespoons sliced almonds
- 1 tablespoon honey (optional)

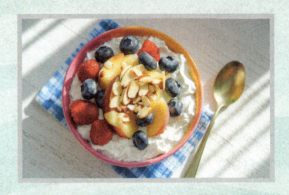

Instructions:

Divide cottage cheese evenly into two bowls. - Top each serving with fresh mixed fruits. - Sprinkle sliced almonds on top. - Drizzle lightly with honey if desired. - Serve immediately.

Nutritional Information (per serving):

Calories: 260 | Protein: 22g | Carbohydrates: 18g | Dietary Fiber: 3g | Sugars: 12g | Fat: 10g (Total), 2g (Saturated) | Cholesterol: 15mg | Sodium: 470mg

avocado and egg toast

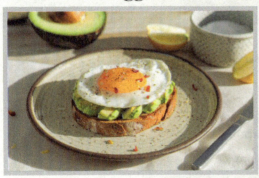

Ingredients (2 servings):

- 2 slices whole-grain bread
- 1 ripe avocado, mashed
- 2 large eggs
- Salt and pepper to taste
- Pinch of red pepper flakes (optional)
- 1 teaspoon olive oil

Instructions:

Toast bread slices until golden and crispy. - Spread mashed avocado evenly on each slice. - Heat olive oil in a non-stick pan over medium heat. - Fry eggs to desired doneness (sunny-side-up or over-easy). - Place one egg on top of each avocado toast slice. - Season with salt, pepper, and red pepper flakes. Serve immediately.

Nutritional Information (per serving - 1 toast):

Calories: 290 | Protein: 12g | Carbohydrates: 18g | Dietary Fiber: 7g | Sugars: 2g | Fat: 19g (Total), 4g (Saturated) | Cholesterol: 185mg | Sodium: 310mg

chia seed protein pudding

Ingredients (2 servings):

- 1½ cups unsweetened almond milk
- ¼ cup chia seeds
- 1 scoop vanilla protein powder (about 25g)
- ½ teaspoon vanilla extract
- ½ cup fresh berries for topping

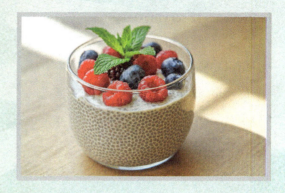

Instructions:

Whisk almond milk, chia seeds, protein powder, and vanilla extract thoroughly in a bowl. - Divide evenly into two serving glasses or bowls. - Refrigerate overnight (or at least 4 hours) until thickened. - Top with fresh berries before serving.

Nutritional Information (per serving):

Calories: 220 | Protein: 15g | Carbohydrates: 16g | Dietary Fiber: 9g | Sugars: 2g | Fat: 10g (Total), 1g (Saturated) | Cholesterol: 0mg | Sodium: 140mg

---

smoked salmon bagel

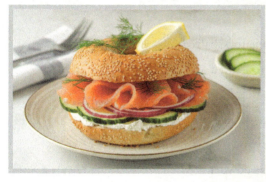

Ingredients (2 servings):

- 2 whole-grain bagels, sliced
- 4 ounces smoked salmon slices
- 4 tablespoons low-fat cream cheese
- ½ cucumber, thinly sliced
- ¼ red onion, thinly sliced
- Fresh dill, for garnish
- Lemon wedges (optional)

Instructions:

Toast bagel slices until lightly crisp. - Spread cream cheese evenly on each half. - Top with smoked salmon slices, cucumber, and red onion. - Garnish with fresh dill and lemon wedges, if desired. - Serve immediately.

Nutritional Information (per serving - 1 bagel):

Calories: 320 | Protein: 20g | Carbohydrates: 34g | Dietary Fiber: 5g | Sugars: 4g | Fat: 11g (Total), 4g (Saturated) | Cholesterol: 30mg | Sodium: 590mg

almond butter banana toast

Ingredients (2 servings):
- 2 slices whole-grain bread
- 4 tablespoons almond butter
- 1 ripe banana, sliced
- 1 tablespoon chia seeds or flax seeds (optional)
- Honey drizzle (optional)

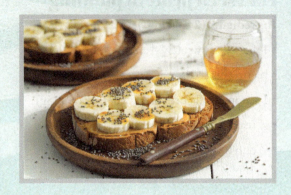

Instructions:

Toast bread slices until golden brown. - Spread almond butter evenly on each slice. - Layer banana slices on top. - Sprinkle chia seeds or flax seeds if using. - Drizzle lightly with honey, if desired. - Serve immediately.

Nutritional Information (per serving - 1 toast):

Calories: 320 | Protein: 10g | Carbohydrates: 31g | Dietary Fiber: 6g | Sugars: 10g | Fat: 16g (Total), 2g (Saturated) | Cholesterol: 0mg | Sodium: 170mg

---

breakfast egg and veggie skillet

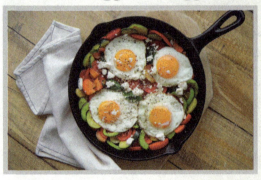

Ingredients (2 servings):
- 4 large eggs
- ½ cup cherry tomatoes, halved
- ½ cup bell peppers, diced
- ½ cup zucchini, diced
- ¼ cup red onion, diced
- 1 tablespoon olive oil
- ¼ teaspoon garlic powder
- Salt and black pepper to taste
- ¼ cup feta cheese, crumbled (optional)

Instructions:

Heat olive oil in a non-stick skillet over medium heat. - Add onion, bell peppers, and zucchini; sauté for 3-4 minutes until softened. - Stir in cherry tomatoes and season with garlic powder, salt, and pepper. - Make four small wells in the vegetable mixture and crack eggs into them. - Cover skillet and cook for 4-5 minutes until egg whites are set but yolks are still runny. - Sprinkle with feta cheese if desired and serve immediately.

Nutritional Information (per serving):

Calories: 280 | Protein: 19g | Carbohydrates: 12g | Dietary Fiber: 3g | Sugars: 6g | Fat: 18g (Total), 5g (Saturated) | Cholesterol: 370mg | Sodium: 320mg

HIGH PROTEIN COOKBOOK

---

berry smoothie bowl

Ingredients (2 servings):

- 1 cup frozen mixed berries
- ½ cup plain Greek yogurt
- ½ cup unsweetened almond milk
- 1 scoop vanilla protein powder (about 25g)
- 1 tablespoon chia seeds
- ¼ cup granola (for topping)
- ¼ cup fresh mixed berries (for topping)

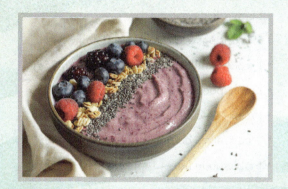

Instructions:

Blend frozen berries, Greek yogurt, almond milk, protein powder, and chia seeds until smooth and creamy. - Divide smoothie mixture evenly into two bowls. - Top with granola and fresh berries. - Serve immediately with a spoon.

Nutritional Information (per serving):

Calories: 290 | Protein: 22g | Carbohydrates: 30g | Dietary Fiber: 7g | Sugars: 14g | Fat: 6g (Total), 1g (Saturated) | Cholesterol: 10mg | Sodium: 80mg

---

turkey sausage and egg muffins

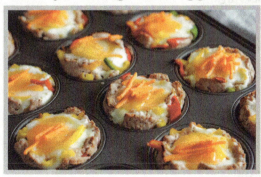

Ingredients (2 servings):

- 4 large eggs
- ½ cup cooked ground turkey sausage
- ¼ cup shredded low-fat cheddar cheese
- ¼ cup diced bell peppers
- ¼ cup diced onions
- ½ teaspoon garlic powder - Salt and pepper to taste - Cooking spray

Instructions:

Preheat oven to 375°F (190°C). - Spray a muffin tin with cooking spray. - In a bowl, whisk eggs, salt, pepper, and garlic powder. - Stir in turkey sausage, bell peppers, onions, and cheese. - Divide mixture evenly into four muffin cups. - Bake for 18-20 minutes or until muffins are firm and golden. - Let cool slightly before serving.

Nutritional Information (per serving - 2 muffins):

Calories: 250 | Protein: 22g | Carbohydrates: 4g | Dietary Fiber: 1g | Sugars: 2g | Fat: 15g (Total), 5g (Saturated) | Cholesterol: 370mg | Sodium: 390mg

overnight protein oats

Ingredients (2 servings):

- 1 cup rolled oats
- 1½ cups unsweetened almond milk
- 1 scoop vanilla protein powder (about 25g)
- 1 tablespoon chia seeds
- 1 teaspoon cinnamon
- ½ cup mixed berries (for topping) -
- 1 tablespoon honey (optional)

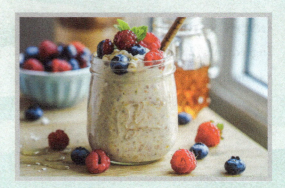

Instructions:

In a mason jar or airtight container, combine oats, almond milk, protein powder, chia seeds, and cinnamon. - Stir well and refrigerate overnight (or for at least 4 hours). - Stir again before serving. - Top with fresh berries and honey if desired. - Serve chilled.

Nutritional Information (per serving):

Calories: 310 | Protein: 22g | Carbohydrates: 40g | Dietary Fiber: 7g | Sugars: 10g | Fat: 7g (Total), 1g (Saturated) | Cholesterol: 0mg | Sodium: 90mg

---

scrambled egg whites with veggies

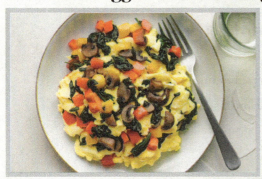

Ingredients (2 servings):

- 6 large egg whites
- ½ cup fresh spinach, chopped
- ¼ cup diced bell peppers
- ¼ cup diced mushrooms
- ¼ teaspoon garlic powder
- Salt and black pepper to taste
- 1 teaspoon olive oil

Instructions:

Heat olive oil in a non-stick skillet over medium heat. - Add bell peppers and mushrooms, sauté for 2 minutes until slightly softened. - Stir in spinach and cook for another minute. - Pour in egg whites and season with salt, pepper, and garlic powder. - Scramble gently until eggs are fully set but still soft. - Serve immediately.

Nutritional Information (per serving):

Calories: 120 | Protein: 20g | Carbohydrates: 5g | Dietary Fiber: 2g | Sugars: 3g | Fat: 2g (Total), 0g (Saturated) | Cholesterol: 0mg | Sodium: 220mg

banana nut protein bread

Ingredients (2 servings):

- 1 large ripe banana, mashed
- ½ cup almond flour
- 1 scoop vanilla protein powder (about 25g)
- 2 large eggs
- ½ teaspoon baking soda
- ¼ teaspoon cinnamon
- 1 tablespoon chopped walnuts - 1 teaspoon honey (optional)

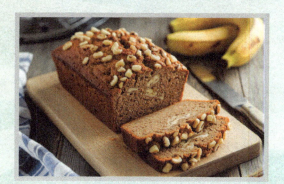

Instructions:

Preheat oven to 350°F (175°C). - In a bowl, mash the banana, then mix in eggs, protein powder, and almond flour. - Stir in baking soda, cinnamon, and walnuts. - Pour batter into a small greased loaf pan. - Bake for 20-25 minutes or until golden brown and a toothpick comes out clean. - Let cool before slicing.

Nutritional Information (per serving - 1 slice):

Calories: 260 | Protein: 18g | Carbohydrates: 22g | Dietary Fiber: 4g | Sugars: 9g | Fat: 12g (Total), 2g (Saturated) | Cholesterol: 125mg | Sodium: 180mg

---

quinoa breakfast bowl

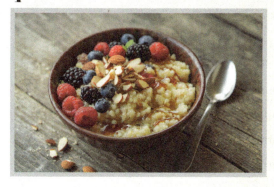

Ingredients (2 servings):

- ½ cup dry quinoa
- 1 cup unsweetened almond milk
- 1 scoop vanilla protein powder (about 25g)
- ½ teaspoon cinnamon
- ½ teaspoon vanilla extract
- ½ cup mixed berries - 1 tablespoon chopped almonds
- 1 teaspoon honey (optional)

Instructions:

Rinse quinoa under cold water. - In a saucepan, combine quinoa and almond milk. Bring to a boil, then reduce heat and simmer for 12-15 minutes, until quinoa is tender. - Stir in protein powder, cinnamon, and vanilla extract. - Divide into two bowls, top with mixed berries and chopped almonds. - Drizzle with honey if desired and serve warm.

Nutritional Information (per serving):

Calories: 280 | Protein: 22g | Carbohydrates: 36g | Dietary Fiber: 5g | Sugars: 8g | Fat: 6g (Total), 1g (Saturated) | Cholesterol: 0mg | Sodium: 75mg

egg and cheese wrap

Ingredients (2 servings):

- 4 large eggs
- ½ cup shredded low-fat cheddar cheese
- 2 whole-wheat tortillas
- ¼ teaspoon garlic powder
- Salt and black pepper to taste
- 1 teaspoon olive oil

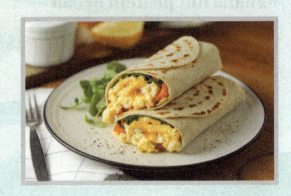

Instructions:

Whisk eggs in a bowl with garlic powder, salt, and pepper. - Heat olive oil in a non-stick pan over medium heat. - Scramble eggs gently until fully cooked but still soft. - Divide eggs evenly onto the tortillas and sprinkle cheese on top. - Roll tortillas into wraps and serve warm.

Nutritional Information (per serving - 1 wrap):

Calories: 320 | Protein: 24g | Carbohydrates: 28g | Dietary Fiber: 5g | Sugars: 2g | Fat: 14g (Total), 5g (Saturated) | Cholesterol: 370mg | Sodium: 410mg

---

tofu scramble

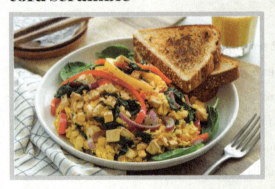

Ingredients (2 servings):

- ½ block firm tofu, crumbled
- 2 Large Eggs
- ½ cup diced bell peppers
- ½ cup baby spinach
- ¼ cup diced onions
- ½ teaspoon turmeric
- ¼ teaspoon garlic powder - ¼ teaspoon black pepper - ½ teaspoon salt - 1 teaspoon olive oil

Instructions:

Heat olive oil in a skillet over medium heat. - Add onions and bell peppers, sauté for 2 minutes. - Stir in crumbled tofu and season with turmeric, garlic powder, salt, and black pepper. - Cook for 3-4 minutes until heated through. Scramble eggs gently until fully cooked but still soft. - Add spinach and cook for an additional minute. - Serve warm.

Nutritional Information (per serving):

Calories: 180 | Protein: 17g | Carbohydrates: 8g | Dietary Fiber: 3g | Sugars: 2g | Fat: 10g (Total), 1g (Saturated) | Cholesterol: 0mg | Sodium: 290mg

protein french toast

Ingredients (2 servings):

- 2 slices whole-grain bread
- 3 large egg whites
- ¼ cup unsweetened almond milk
- ½ scoop vanilla protein powder (about 12g)
- ½ teaspoon cinnamon
- ½ teaspoon vanilla extract
- ½ teaspoon coconut oil
- ½ cup fresh berries (for topping)

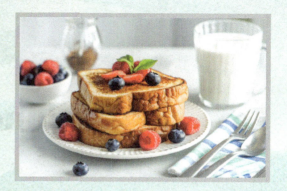

Instructions:

In a shallow bowl, whisk egg whites, almond milk, protein powder, cinnamon, and vanilla extract. - Dip each slice of bread into the mixture, coating evenly. - Heat coconut oil in a pan over medium heat. - Cook bread slices for 2-3 minutes per side until golden brown. - Serve warm, topped with fresh berries.

Nutritional Information (per serving):

Calories: 180 | Protein: 17g | Carbohydrates: 8g | Dietary Fiber: 3g | Sugars: 2g | Fat: 10g (Total), 1g (Saturated) | Cholesterol: 0mg | Sodium: 290mg

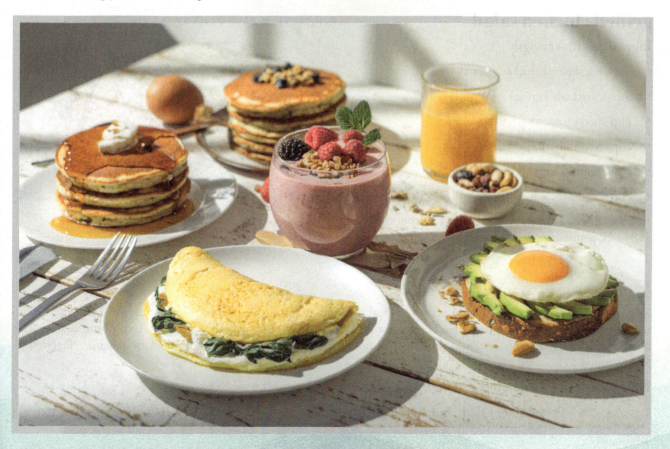

lunch recipes

...

Energize Your Afternoons

A high-protein lunch is essential to keep your energy levels steady, prevent afternoon crashes, and support muscle maintenance while losing weight. These easy, nutrient-dense recipes will help you stay full, satisfied, and on track with your health goals.

grilled chicken salad

Ingredients (2 servings):

- 2 boneless, skinless chicken breasts
- 4 cups mixed salad greens
- ½ cup cherry tomatoes, halved
- ¼ cup red onion, thinly sliced
- ¼ cup crumbled feta cheese
- ¼ cup sliced almonds
- 2 tablespoons balsamic vinaigrette - 1 teaspoon olive oil - Salt and black pepper to taste

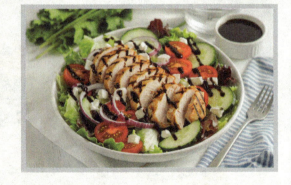

Instructions:

Season chicken breasts with salt and pepper. - Heat olive oil in a grill pan over medium heat. - Grill chicken for 5-6 minutes per side, until fully cooked. - Let rest for 5 minutes before slicing. - In a large bowl, combine salad greens, cherry tomatoes, red onion, feta, and almonds. - Top with grilled chicken slices and drizzle with balsamic vinaigrette. - Serve immediately.

Nutritional Information (per serving):

Calories: 350 | Protein: 40g | Carbohydrates: 10g | Dietary Fiber: 3g | Sugars: 4g | Fat: 14g (Total), 3g (Saturated) | Cholesterol: 90mg | Sodium: 400mg

tuna avocado wrap

Ingredients (2 servings):

- 1 can (5 oz) tuna, drained
- 1 ripe avocado, mashed
- ¼ cup Greek yogurt (plain, non-fat)
- ½ teaspoon garlic powder
- ½ teaspoon lemon juice
- Salt and black pepper to taste
- 2 whole-wheat tortillas - ½ cup baby spinach

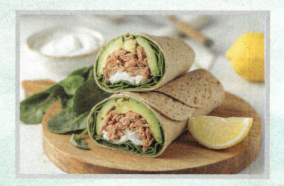

Instructions:

In a bowl, mash avocado and mix with tuna, Greek yogurt, garlic powder, lemon juice, salt, and pepper. - Spread the mixture evenly on whole-wheat tortillas. - Layer with baby spinach leaves. - Roll tortillas tightly into wraps. - Slice in half and serve.

Nutritional Information (per serving - 1 wrap):

Calories: 320 | Protein: 28g | Carbohydrates: 28g | Dietary Fiber: 6g | Sugars: 2g | Fat: 12g (Total), 2g (Saturated) | Cholesterol: 35mg | Sodium: 480mg

---

quinoa and chickpea bowl

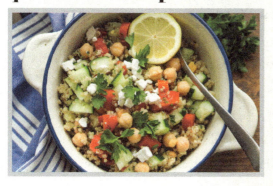

Ingredients (2 servings):

- ½ cup dry quinoa - 1 cup of water
- ½ cup canned chickpeas, drained and rinsed
- ½ cup diced cucumber
- ¼ cup diced red bell pepper
- ¼ cup crumbled feta cheese
- 2 tablespoons lemon juice - 1 teaspoon olive oil
- ½ teaspoon cumin - Salt and black pepper to taste

Instructions:

Rinse quinoa under cold water. - In a saucepan, bring quinoa and water to a boil. Reduce heat, cover, and simmer for 12-15 minutes until quinoa is tender. - In a large bowl, mix quinoa with chickpeas, cucumber, red bell pepper, and feta cheese. - Drizzle with lemon juice, olive oil, and sprinkle with cumin, salt, and black pepper. - Toss well and serve.

Nutritional Information (per serving):

Calories: 280 | Protein: 16g | Carbohydrates: 38g | Dietary Fiber: 7g | Sugars: 3g | Fat: 9g (Total), 2g (Saturated) | Cholesterol: 10mg | Sodium: 320mg

high protein cobb salad

Ingredients (2 servings):

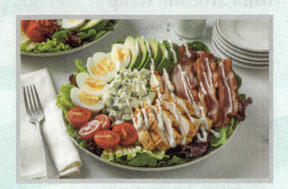

- 2 boneless, skinless chicken breasts, grilled and sliced
- 4 cups romaine lettuce, chopped
- 2 hard-boiled eggs, sliced
- ½ avocado, diced
- ½ cup cherry tomatoes, halved
- ¼ cup crumbled blue cheese
- 2 slices turkey bacon, cooked and crumbled - 2 tablespoons ranch dressing (light)

Instructions:

Season and grill chicken, then slice. - Arrange lettuce in two bowls. - Top with eggs, avocado, cherry tomatoes, blue cheese, and turkey bacon. - Add grilled chicken slices. - Drizzle with ranch dressing and serve.

Nutritional Information (per serving):

Calories: 420 | Protein: 45g | Carbohydrates: 12g | Dietary Fiber: 5g | Sugars: 3g | Fat: 20g (Total), 6g (Saturated) | Cholesterol: 290mg | Sodium: 520mg

---

turkey and veggie sandwich

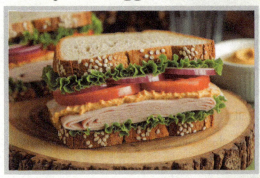

Ingredients (2 servings):

- 4 slices whole-wheat bread
- 6 ounces deli turkey breast, low sodium
- 4 lettuce leaves
- 4 tomato slices
- ¼ red onion, thinly sliced
- 2 tablespoons hummus - ½ teaspoon Dijon mustard

Instructions:

Spread hummus on two slices of whole-wheat bread. - Spread Dijon mustard on the other two slices. - Layer lettuce, turkey, tomato, and onion on hummus-covered bread. - Top with the other bread slices. - Cut in half and serve.

Nutritional Information (per serving - 1 sandwich):

Calories: 310 | Protein: 30g | Carbohydrates: 35g | Dietary Fiber: 6g | Sugars: 4g | Fat: 6g (Total), 1g (Saturated) | Cholesterol: 35mg | Sodium: 450mg

lentil soup

Ingredients (2 servings):

- ½ cup dry lentils, rinsed
- 2 cups low-sodium vegetable broth
- ½ cup diced carrots
- ½ cup diced celery
- ¼ cup diced onion
- 1 clove garlic, minced
- 1 teaspoon olive oil - ½ teaspoon cumin - ¼ teaspoon black pepper
- ¼ teaspoon salt

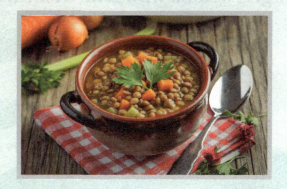

Instructions:

Heat olive oil in a pot over medium heat. - Add onion, carrots, and celery, sauté for 3-4 minutes until softened. - Stir in garlic, cumin, salt, and pepper, cook for another minute. - Add lentils and vegetable broth, bring to a boil. - Reduce heat, cover, and simmer for 25-30 minutes until lentils are tender. - Serve warm.

Nutritional Information (per serving):

Calories: 280 | Protein: 20g | Carbohydrates: 38g | Dietary Fiber: 14g | Sugars: 4g | Fat: 5g (Total), 1g (Saturated) | Cholesterol: 0mg | Sodium: 300mg

---

chicken caesar wrap

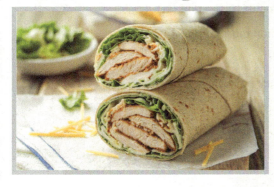

Ingredients (2 servings):

- 6 ounces grilled chicken breast, sliced
- 2 whole-wheat tortillas
- 2 cups chopped romaine lettuce
- ¼ cup shredded Parmesan cheese
- 2 tablespoons light Caesar dressing
- ¼ teaspoon black pepper

Instructions:

In a bowl, mix romaine lettuce, Parmesan cheese, black pepper, and Caesar dressing. - Place an even amount of grilled chicken on each tortilla. - Top with dressed lettuce mixture. - Roll tortillas tightly into wraps. - Slice in half and serve.

Nutritional Information (per serving - 1 wrap):

Calories: 350 | Protein: 38g | Carbohydrates: 28g | Dietary Fiber: 4g | Sugars: 2g | Fat: 10g (Total), 3g (Saturated) | Cholesterol: 85mg | Sodium: 480mg

greek salad with grilled chicken

Ingredients (2 servings):

- 6 ounces grilled chicken breast, sliced
- 4 cups romaine lettuce, chopped
- ½ cup cherry tomatoes, halved
- ¼ cup sliced cucumber
- ¼ cup crumbled feta cheese
- ¼ cup sliced Kalamata olives
- 2 tablespoons lemon vinaigrette

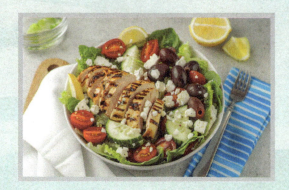

Instructions:

In a large bowl, combine romaine lettuce, cherry tomatoes, cucumber, feta, and olives. - Add grilled chicken slices on top. - Drizzle with lemon vinaigrette and toss gently. - Serve immediately.

Nutritional Information (per serving):

Calories: 360 | Protein: 42g | Carbohydrates: 10g | Dietary Fiber: 4g | Sugars: 3g | Fat: 14g (Total), 4g (Saturated) | Cholesterol: 95mg | Sodium: 420mg

---

egg salad lettuce wraps

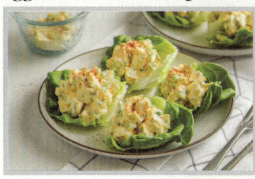

Ingredients (2 servings):

- 4 hard-boiled eggs, chopped
- ¼ cup Greek yogurt (plain, non-fat)
- ½ teaspoon Dijon mustard
- ¼ teaspoon salt
- ¼ teaspoon black pepper
- ½ teaspoon paprika
- 4 large romaine lettuce leaves

Instructions:

In a bowl, mix chopped eggs, Greek yogurt, Dijon mustard, salt, black pepper, and paprika until well combined. - Spoon egg salad evenly onto lettuce leaves. - Roll or fold leaves to form wraps. - Serve immediately.

Nutritional Information (per serving - 2 lettuce wraps):

Calories: 220 | Protein: 18g | Carbohydrates: 5g | Dietary Fiber: 2g | Sugars: 2g | Fat: 14g (Total), 4g (Saturated) | Cholesterol: 375mg | Sodium: 350mg

salmon sushi bowl

Ingredients (2 servings):

- 6 ounces fresh salmon, diced
- 1 cup cooked brown rice
- ½ cup cucumber, diced
- ½ avocado, sliced
- ¼ cup shredded carrots
- 1 tablespoon low-sodium soy sauce
- 1 teaspoon sesame seeds - 1 teaspoon rice vinegar

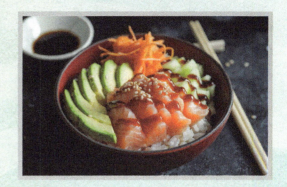

Instructions:

In two bowls, divide cooked brown rice evenly. - Top with diced salmon, cucumber, avocado, and shredded carrots. - Drizzle with soy sauce and rice vinegar. - Sprinkle sesame seeds on top and serve.

Nutritional Information (per serving):

Calories: 420 | Protein: 42g | Carbohydrates: 36g | Dietary Fiber: 6g | Sugars: 3g | Fat: 15g (Total), 4g (Saturated) | Cholesterol: 85mg | Sodium: 420mg

---

black bean burrito bowl

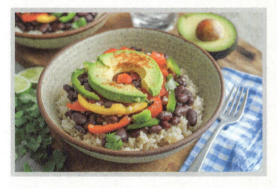

Ingredients (2 servings):

- 1 cup cooked brown rice
- ½ cup canned black beans, drained and rinsed
- ½ cup diced bell peppers
- ½ cup cherry tomatoes, halved
- ¼ cup diced red onion
- ½ avocado, sliced
- ¼ teaspoon cumin
- ¼ teaspoon chili powder - 1 teaspoon olive oil - Salt and black pepper to taste

Instructions:

Heat olive oil in a pan over medium heat. - Add bell peppers and red onion, sauté for 3 minutes. - Stir in black beans, cumin, chili powder, salt, and pepper, cook for another 2 minutes. - Divide brown rice into two bowls. - Top with sautéed black bean mixture, cherry tomatoes, and avocado slices. - Serve warm.

Nutritional Information (per serving):

Calories: 380 | Protein: 18g | Carbohydrates: 45g | Dietary Fiber: 10g | Sugars: 6g | Fat: 12g (Total), 2g (Saturated) | Cholesterol: 0mg | Sodium: 320mg

chicken fajita salad

Ingredients (2 servings):

- 6 ounces grilled chicken breast, sliced
- 4 cups mixed salad greens
- ½ cup sliced bell peppers
- ¼ cup diced red onion
- ¼ cup shredded low-fat cheddar cheese
- 2 tablespoons Greek yogurt (for dressing)
- ½ teaspoon smoked paprika - ½ teaspoon cumin - 1 teaspoon olive oil - Salt and black pepper to taste

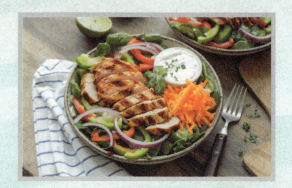

Instructions:

Heat olive oil in a pan over medium heat. - Add bell peppers, red onion, smoked paprika, and cumin, sauté for 3 minutes. - Arrange salad greens in two bowls. - Top with grilled chicken slices, sautéed veggies, and shredded cheddar. - Drizzle with Greek yogurt and serve.

Nutritional Information (per serving):

Calories: 340 | Protein: 42g | Carbohydrates: 12g | Dietary Fiber: 4g | Sugars: 3g | Fat: 12g (Total), 4g (Saturated) | Cholesterol: 95mg | Sodium: 410mg

protein pasta primavera

Ingredients (2 servings):

- 4 ounces whole-wheat pasta - ½ cup diced zucchini
- ½ cup cherry tomatoes, halved - ¼ cup diced bell peppers
- ¼ cup shredded Parmesan cheese - ½ teaspoon garlic powder
- ½ teaspoon oregano - 1 teaspoon olive oil - 6 ounces grilled chicken breast, sliced - Salt and black pepper to taste

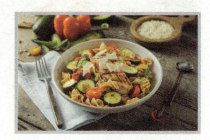

Instructions:

Cook whole-wheat pasta according to package instructions. - Heat olive oil in a pan over medium heat. - Add zucchini, bell peppers, and cherry tomatoes, sauté for 3 minutes. - Stir in garlic powder, oregano, salt, and pepper. - Mix with cooked pasta and grilled chicken. - Top with Parmesan cheese and serve warm.

Nutritional Information (per serving):

Calories: 420 | Protein: 42g | Carbohydrates: 48g | Dietary Fiber: 8g | Sugars: 6g | Fat: 10g (Total), 3g (Saturated) | Cholesterol: 90mg | Sodium: 380mg

shrimp and quinoa salad

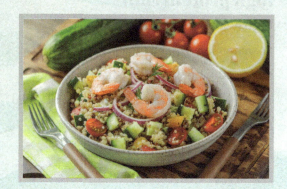

Ingredients (2 servings):

- ½ cup dry quinoa
- 1 cup water
- 8 ounces shrimp, peeled and deveined
- ½ cup diced cucumber
- ½ cup cherry tomatoes, halved
- ¼ cup diced red onion
- 2 tablespoons lemon juice - 1 teaspoon olive oil - ¼ teaspoon black pepper - ¼ teaspoon salt

Instructions:

Rinse quinoa under cold water. - In a saucepan, bring quinoa and water to a boil. Reduce heat, cover, and simmer for 12-15 minutes. - Heat olive oil in a pan over medium heat. - Add shrimp, season with salt and pepper, and cook for 3-4 minutes per side. - In a bowl, mix quinoa, cucumber, cherry tomatoes, and red onion. - Top with cooked shrimp, drizzle with lemon juice, and serve.

Nutritional Information (per serving):

Calories: 380 | Protein: 40g | Carbohydrates: 34g | Dietary Fiber: 5g | Sugars: 4g | Fat: 10g (Total), 2g (Saturated) | Cholesterol: 200mg | Sodium: 420mg

---

avocado chicken wrap

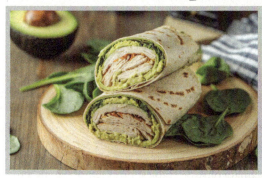

Ingredients (2 servings):

- 6 ounces grilled chicken breast, sliced
- 2 whole-wheat tortillas
- 1 ripe avocado, mashed
- ½ cup baby spinach
- ¼ teaspoon garlic powder - Salt and black pepper to taste - 1 teaspoon olive oil

Instructions:

Mash avocado in a bowl, season with garlic powder, salt, and pepper. - Spread mashed avocado evenly onto each tortilla. - Layer with spinach and grilled chicken slices. - Roll tortillas tightly into wraps. - Slice in half and serve.

Nutritional Information (per serving - 1 wrap):

Calories: 380 | Protein: 36g | Carbohydrates: 28g | Dietary Fiber: 6g | Sugars: 2g | Fat: 15g (Total), 3g (Saturated) | Cholesterol: 90mg | Sodium: 410mg

high protein chili

Ingredients (2 servings):

- 6 ounces lean ground turkey
- ½ cup canned black beans, drained and rinsed
- ½ cup canned kidney beans, drained and rinsed
- 1 cup diced tomatoes
- ½ cup diced bell peppers
- ¼ cup diced onions
- 1 teaspoon olive oil
- 1 teaspoon chili powder - ½ teaspoon cumin - ¼ teaspoon garlic powder - ¼ teaspoon salt - 1 cup low-sodium chicken broth

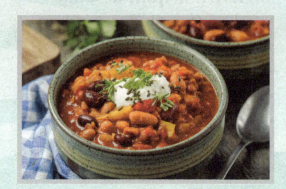

Instructions:

Heat olive oil in a large pot over medium heat. - Add onions and bell peppers, sauté for 3 minutes. - Stir in ground turkey, breaking it up with a spoon, and cook until browned. - Add beans, diced tomatoes, chili powder, cumin, garlic powder, salt, and chicken broth. - Bring to a boil, then reduce heat and let simmer for 20-25 minutes. - Serve warm.

Nutritional Information (per serving):

Calories: 420 | Protein: 45g | Carbohydrates: 36g | Dietary Fiber: 10g | Sugars: 6g | Fat: 10g (Total), 3g (Saturated) | Cholesterol: 85mg | Sodium: 400mg

---

mediterranean chicken bowl

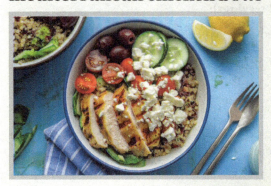

Ingredients (2 servings):

- 6 ounces grilled chicken breast, sliced
- ½ cup cooked quinoa
- ½ cup diced cucumber
- ¼ cup cherry tomatoes, halved
- ¼ cup crumbled feta cheese
- ¼ cup sliced Kalamata olives - 2 tablespoons lemon vinaigrette

Instructions:

In two bowls, divide cooked quinoa evenly. - Top with grilled chicken, diced cucumber, cherry tomatoes, feta, and olives. - Drizzle with lemon vinaigrette. - Serve immediately.

Nutritional Information (per serving):

Calories: 380 | Protein: 42g | Carbohydrates: 30g | Dietary Fiber: 6g | Sugars: 4g | Fat: 12g (Total), 3g (Saturated) | Cholesterol: 90mg | Sodium: 450mg

asian tofu salad

Ingredients (2 servings):

- 6 ounces firm tofu, cubed
- 4 cups mixed greens
- ½ cup shredded carrots
- ¼ cup sliced red bell peppers - ¼ cup edamame beans
- 1 teaspoon sesame oil - 1 tablespoon low-sodium soy sauce
- 1 teaspoon rice vinegar - ½ teaspoon sesame seeds

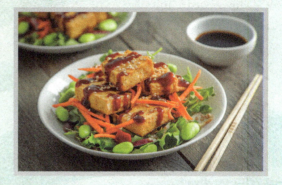

Instructions:

Heat sesame oil in a pan over medium heat. - Add tofu cubes and cook until golden brown, about 5 minutes. - In a large bowl, combine mixed greens, carrots, red bell peppers, and edamame. - Top with crispy tofu. - Drizzle with soy sauce and rice vinegar, then sprinkle sesame seeds. - Serve immediately.

Nutritional Information (per serving):

Calories: 320 | Protein: 30g | Carbohydrates: 22g | Dietary Fiber: 6g | Sugars: 4g | Fat: 14g (Total), 2g (Saturated) | Cholesterol: 0mg | Sodium: 400mg

---

turkey burger lettuce wrap

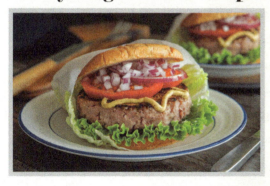

Ingredients (2 servings):

- 6 ounces lean ground turkey
- ¼ teaspoon garlic powder
- ¼ teaspoon onion powder
- ¼ teaspoon black pepper
- ¼ teaspoon salt
- 4 large romaine lettuce leaves - ¼ cup sliced tomatoes
- ¼ cup diced red onion - 1 teaspoon Dijon mustard

Instructions:

Preheat a grill or skillet over medium heat. - In a bowl, mix ground turkey with garlic powder, onion powder, black pepper, and salt. - Form into two patties. - Cook for 4-5 minutes per side until fully cooked. - Serve patties wrapped in lettuce leaves with tomato slices, diced onions, and a drizzle of Dijon mustard.

Nutritional Information (per serving - 1 lettuce wrap):

Calories: 280 | Protein: 38g | Carbohydrates: 6g | Dietary Fiber: 2g | Sugars: 2g | Fat: 12g (Total), 3g (Saturated) | Cholesterol: 90mg | Sodium: 350mg

lentil and veggie stir-fry

Ingredients (2 servings):

- ½ cup cooked lentils
- ½ cup diced zucchini
- ½ cup diced bell peppers
- ¼ cup sliced mushrooms
- 1 teaspoon olive oil
- 1 teaspoon low-sodium soy sauce
- ½ teaspoon garlic powder - ¼ teaspoon black pepper
- ¼ teaspoon salt

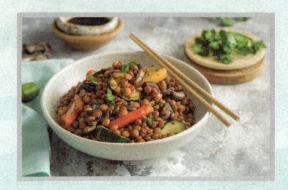

Instructions:

Heat olive oil in a pan over medium heat. - Add zucchini, bell peppers, and mushrooms, sauté for 3 minutes. - Stir in cooked lentils, soy sauce, garlic powder, black pepper, and salt. - Cook for another 2-3 minutes. - Serve warm.

Nutritional Information (per serving):

Calories: 290 | Protein: 22g | Carbohydrates: 35g | Dietary Fiber: 9g | Sugars: 5g | Fat: 6g (Total), 1g (Saturated) | Cholesterol: 0mg | Sodium: 350mg

---

salmon avocado salad

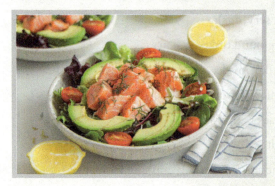

Ingredients (2 servings):

- 6 ounces cooked salmon, flaked
- 4 cups mixed greens
- ½ avocado, diced
- ½ cup cherry tomatoes, halved
- ¼ cup diced cucumber
- 2 tablespoons lemon vinaigrette - 1 teaspoon olive oil
- ¼ teaspoon black pepper - ¼ teaspoon salt

Instructions:

In a large bowl, combine mixed greens, cherry tomatoes, cucumber, and diced avocado. - Flake cooked salmon into bite-sized pieces and add to the salad. - Drizzle with lemon vinaigrette and olive oil. - Toss gently and serve immediately.

Nutritional Information (per serving):

Calories: 380 | Protein: 42g | Carbohydrates: 10g | Dietary Fiber: 5g | Sugars: 3g | Fat: 18g (Total), 5g (Saturated) | Cholesterol: 85mg | Sodium: 420mg

chickpea protein wrap

Ingredients (2 servings):

- 1 cup canned chickpeas, drained and rinsed
- ¼ cup diced red bell pepper
- ¼ cup diced cucumber
- ¼ cup shredded carrots
- 2 whole-wheat tortillas
- 2 tablespoons hummus
- ¼ teaspoon garlic powder - ¼ teaspoon black pepper - ½ teaspoon lemon juice

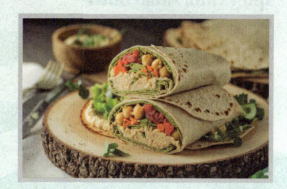

Instructions:

Mash chickpeas in a bowl until slightly chunky. - Mix in diced bell pepper, cucumber, shredded carrots, garlic powder, black pepper, and lemon juice. - Spread hummus evenly on tortillas. - Divide the chickpea mixture evenly between tortillas. - Roll tightly into wraps and serve.

Nutritional Information (per serving - 1 wrap):

Calories: 350 | Protein: 22g | Carbohydrates: 42g | Dietary Fiber: 9g | Sugars: 4g | Fat: 10g (Total), 1g (Saturated) | Cholesterol: 0mg | Sodium: 360mg

---

spinach & turkey meatballs

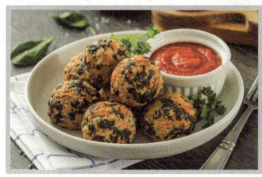

Ingredients (2 servings):

- 6 ounces lean ground turkey
- ½ cup fresh spinach, finely chopped
- ¼ cup whole-wheat breadcrumbs
- 1 egg
- ¼ teaspoon garlic powder
- ¼ teaspoon black pepper - ¼ teaspoon salt - 1 teaspoon olive oil

Instructions:

Preheat oven to 375°F (190°C). - In a bowl, mix ground turkey, spinach, breadcrumbs, egg, garlic powder, salt, and black pepper. - Form into small meatballs. - Heat olive oil in a pan over medium heat, then brown meatballs on all sides. - Transfer to a baking sheet and bake for 10-12 minutes. - Serve warm.

Nutritional Information (per serving - 3-4 meatballs):

Calories: 320 | Protein: 42g | Carbohydrates: 10g | Dietary Fiber: 2g | Sugars: 1g | Fat: 14g (Total), 4g (Saturated) | Cholesterol: 125mg | Sodium: 420mg

spicy tuna salad bowl

Ingredients (2 servings):
- 1 can (5 oz) tuna, drained
- ½ avocado, mashed
- ¼ cup diced red onion
- ½ teaspoon sriracha sauce
- ½ teaspoon lemon juice
- ¼ teaspoon black pepper
- ½ cup cooked quinoa - 4 cups mixed greens

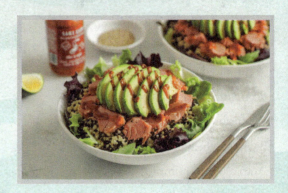

Instructions:

In a bowl, mix tuna, mashed avocado, red onion, sriracha sauce, lemon juice, and black pepper. - Divide mixed greens into two serving bowls. - Add cooked quinoa and top with tuna mixture. - Serve immediately.

Nutritional Information (per serving):

Calories: 360 | Protein: 40g | Carbohydrates: 24g | Dietary Fiber: 6g | Sugars: 2g | Fat: 14g (Total), 2g (Saturated) | Cholesterol: 40mg | Sodium: 420mg

---

veggie omelette wrap

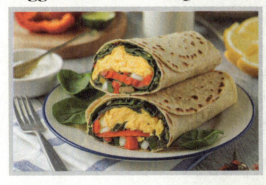

Ingredients (2 servings):
- 4 large eggs
- ½ cup diced bell peppers
- ½ cup baby spinach
- ¼ cup diced onions
- ¼ teaspoon garlic powder
- Salt and black pepper to taste
- 1 teaspoon olive oil
- 2 whole-wheat tortillas

Instructions:

Whisk eggs in a bowl with garlic powder, salt, and pepper. - Heat olive oil in a skillet over medium heat. - Add onions and bell peppers, sauté for 2 minutes. - Pour in whisked eggs and cook until set. - Stir in spinach and cook for another minute. - Divide the mixture between two tortillas and wrap tightly. - Serve warm.

Nutritional Information (per serving - 1 wrap):

Calories: 350 | Protein: 28g | Carbohydrates: 28g | Dietary Fiber: 6g | Sugars: 3g | Fat: 14g (Total), 4g (Saturated) | Cholesterol: 370mg | Sodium: 380mg

high protein buddha bowl

Ingredients (2 servings):

- ½ cup cooked quinoa
- 6 ounces grilled chicken breast, sliced
- ½ cup roasted sweet potatoes, diced
- ½ cup steamed broccoli florets
- ½ avocado, sliced
- 2 tablespoons hummus
- 1 teaspoon olive oil - ¼ teaspoon black pepper - ¼ teaspoon salt

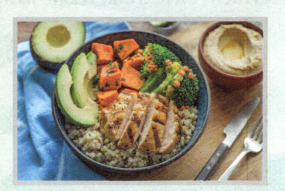

Instructions:

Divide cooked quinoa between two bowls. - Arrange grilled chicken, roasted sweet potatoes, steamed broccoli, and avocado slices on top. - Drizzle with olive oil and season with salt and pepper. - Add a dollop of hummus to each bowl. - Serve immediately.

Nutritional Information (per serving):

Calories: 420 | Protein: 42g | Carbohydrates: 34g | Dietary Fiber: 8g | Sugars: 6g | Fat: 14g (Total), 3g (Saturated) | Cholesterol: 90mg | Sodium: 360mg

---

egg and tuna salad

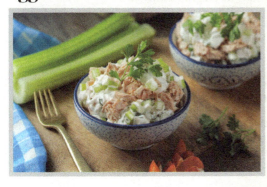

Ingredients (2 servings):

- 2 hard-boiled eggs, chopped
- 1 can (5 oz) tuna, drained
- ¼ cup Greek yogurt (plain, non-fat)
- ½ teaspoon Dijon mustard
- ¼ teaspoon black pepper
- ¼ teaspoon salt
- ½ teaspoon lemon juice - ½ cup diced celery

Instructions:

In a bowl, mix chopped eggs, tuna, Greek yogurt, Dijon mustard, black pepper, salt, and lemon juice. - Stir in diced celery. - Serve in a bowl or as a filling for lettuce wraps.

Nutritional Information (per serving):

Calories: 320 | Protein: 38g | Carbohydrates: 6g | Dietary Fiber: 2g | Sugars: 1g | Fat: 14g (Total), 3g (Saturated) | Cholesterol: 230mg | Sodium: 380mg

grilled chicken and veggie wrap

Ingredients (2 servings):

- 6 ounces grilled chicken breast, sliced
- 2 whole-wheat tortillas
- ½ cup baby spinach
- ¼ cup shredded carrots
- ¼ cup diced bell peppers
- 1 tablespoon hummus - ¼ teaspoon garlic powder - Salt and black pepper to taste

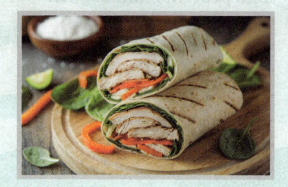

Instructions:

Spread hummus evenly on each tortilla. - Layer with spinach, shredded carrots, diced bell peppers, and grilled chicken. - Sprinkle with garlic powder, salt, and black pepper. - Roll tightly into wraps. - Slice in half and serve.

Nutritional Information (per serving - 1 wrap):

Calories: 350 | Protein: 38g | Carbohydrates: 28g | Dietary Fiber: 6g | Sugars: 3g | Fat: 10g (Total), 2g (Saturated) | Cholesterol: 85mg | Sodium: 400mg

---

steak salad with protein dressing

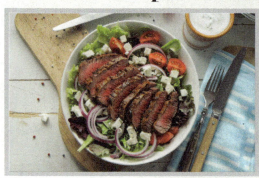

Ingredients (2 servings):

- 6 ounces lean sirloin steak, grilled and sliced
- 4 cups mixed salad greens
- ½ cup cherry tomatoes, halved
- ¼ cup diced cucumber
- ¼ cup red onion, thinly sliced
- ¼ cup crumbled feta cheese
- 2 tablespoons Greek yogurt (for dressing)
- 1 teaspoon olive oil - ¼ teaspoon black pepper - ¼ teaspoon salt

Instructions:

Grill steak to desired doneness and slice thinly. - In a large bowl, combine salad greens, cherry tomatoes, cucumber, and red onion. - Top with steak slices and crumbled feta. - Mix Greek yogurt with olive oil, salt, and black pepper for dressing. - Drizzle dressing over salad and serve.

Nutritional Information (per serving):

Calories: 410 | Protein: 44g | Carbohydrates: 12g | Dietary Fiber: 4g | Sugars: 3g | Fat: 18g (Total), 5g (Saturated) | Cholesterol: 90mg | Sodium: 420mg

protein-packed turkey soup

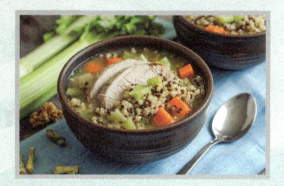

Ingredients (2 servings):
- 6 ounces lean ground turkey
- 2 cups low-sodium chicken broth
- ½ cup diced carrots
- ½ cup diced celery
- ¼ cup diced onion
- 1 clove garlic, minced
- ½ teaspoon dried thyme
- ½ teaspoon black pepper - 1 teaspoon olive oil - ½ cup cooked quinoa

Instructions:

Heat olive oil in a pot over medium heat. - Add onion, carrots, celery, and garlic, sauté for 3 minutes. - Add ground turkey and cook until browned. - Stir in chicken broth, thyme, and black pepper. - Simmer for 15 minutes. - Add cooked quinoa and serve warm.

Nutritional Information (per serving):

Calories: 380 | Protein: 45g | Carbohydrates: 28g | Dietary Fiber: 6g | Sugars: 4g | Fat: 10g (Total), 2g (Saturated) | Cholesterol: 85mg | Sodium: 420mg

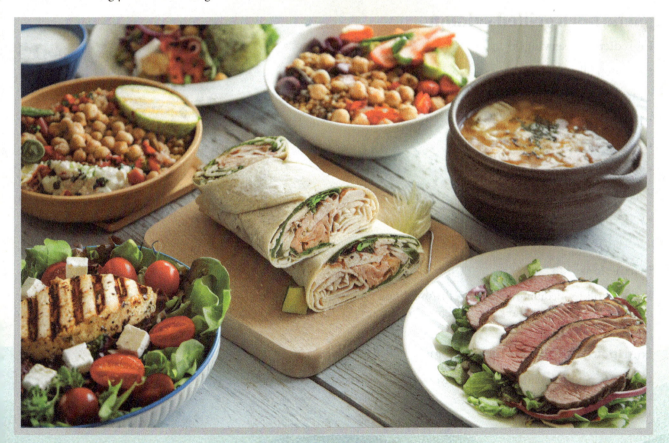

dinner recipes

. . .

Healthy Meals to Satisfy and Sustain

Dinner is the perfect opportunity to refuel your body with nutrient-dense, high-protein meals that promote muscle recovery and weight loss. These recipes are designed to be satisfying, packed with lean protein, and easy to prepare in under 30 minutes.

garlic herb grilled salmon

Ingredients (2 servings):

- 2 salmon fillets (6 oz each)
- 1 teaspoon olive oil
- 1 teaspoon lemon juice
- ½ teaspoon garlic powder
- ½ teaspoon dried oregano
- ¼ teaspoon black pepper
- ¼ teaspoon salt

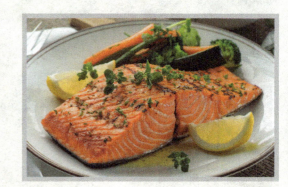

Instructions:

Preheat grill to medium-high heat. - Brush salmon fillets with olive oil and lemon juice. - Season with garlic powder, oregano, black pepper, and salt. - Grill for 4-5 minutes per side until flaky. - Serve hot with steamed vegetables or a side salad.

Nutritional Information (per serving):

Calories: 380 | Protein: 42g | Carbohydrates: 2g | Dietary Fiber: 0g | Sugars: 0g | Fat: 20g (Total), 5g (Saturated) | Cholesterol: 85mg | Sodium: 320mg

chicken and broccoli stir-fry

Ingredients (2 servings):

- 6 ounces chicken breast, sliced
- 2 cups broccoli florets
- ½ cup sliced bell peppers
- 1 teaspoon olive oil
- 1 teaspoon low-sodium soy sauce
- ½ teaspoon garlic powder - ½ teaspoon ginger powder
- ¼ teaspoon black pepper

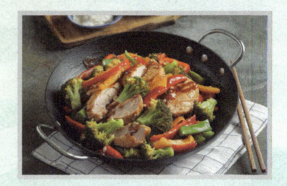

Instructions:

Heat olive oil in a skillet over medium heat. - Add chicken slices and cook for 4-5 minutes until browned. - Stir in broccoli, bell peppers, soy sauce, garlic powder, ginger powder, and black pepper. - Cook for another 5 minutes until vegetables are tender. - Serve warm.

Nutritional Information (per serving):

Calories: 320 | Protein: 40g | Carbohydrates: 12g | Dietary Fiber: 4g | Sugars: 4g | Fat: 8g (Total), 2g (Saturated) | Cholesterol: 85mg | Sodium: 420mg

---

protein-rich turkey meatloaf

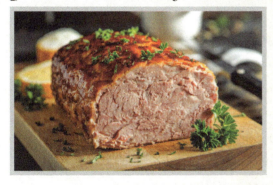

Ingredients (2 servings):

- 6 ounces lean ground turkey
- ¼ cup whole-wheat breadcrumbs
- 1 egg
- ½ teaspoon garlic powder
- ½ teaspoon onion powder
- ½ teaspoon dried oregano
- ¼ teaspoon black pepper - ¼ teaspoon salt

Instructions:

Preheat oven to 375°F (190°C). - In a bowl, mix ground turkey, breadcrumbs, egg, garlic powder, onion powder, oregano, black pepper, and salt. - Shape into a small loaf and place in a greased baking dish. - Bake for 25-30 minutes until cooked through. - Let rest for 5 minutes before slicing.

Nutritional Information (per serving):

Calories: 340 | Protein: 42g | Carbohydrates: 10g | Dietary Fiber: 2g | Sugars: 1g | Fat: 12g (Total), 3g (Saturated) | Cholesterol: 125mg | Sodium: 420mg

steak with grilled vegetables

Ingredients (2 servings):

- 6 ounces lean sirloin steak
- 1 teaspoon olive oil
- ½ teaspoon garlic powder
- ¼ teaspoon black pepper
- ¼ teaspoon salt
- ½ cup sliced zucchini
- ½ cup sliced bell peppers
- ½ cup asparagus spears

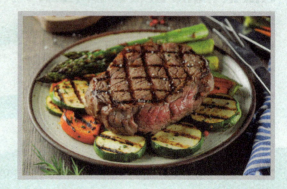

Instructions:

Preheat grill to medium-high heat. - Rub steak with olive oil, garlic powder, black pepper, and salt. - Grill steak for 4-5 minutes per side to desired doneness. - Grill vegetables for 3-4 minutes until tender. - Serve steak with grilled vegetables on the side.

Nutritional Information (per serving):

Calories: 420 | Protein: 46g | Carbohydrates: 10g | Dietary Fiber: 4g | Sugars: 4g | Fat: 18g (Total), 6g (Saturated) | Cholesterol: 90mg | Sodium: 400mg

---

oven-baked cod with herbs

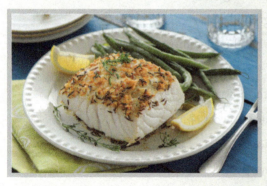

Ingredients (2 servings):

- 2 cod fillets (6 oz each)
- 1 teaspoon olive oil
- ½ teaspoon lemon juice
- ½ teaspoon dried thyme
- ¼ teaspoon garlic powder
- ¼ teaspoon salt - ¼ teaspoon black pepper

Instructions:

Preheat oven to 375°F (190°C). - Place cod fillets on a baking sheet lined with parchment paper. - Drizzle with olive oil and lemon juice. - Season with thyme, garlic powder, salt, and black pepper. - Bake for 12-15 minutes until flaky. - Serve warm.

Nutritional Information (per serving):

Calories: 280 | Protein: 38g | Carbohydrates: 2g | Dietary Fiber: 0g | Sugars: 0g | Fat: 12g (Total), 2g (Saturated) | Cholesterol: 70mg | Sodium: 320mg

chicken quinoa bowl

Ingredients (2 servings):

- 6 ounces grilled chicken breast, sliced
- ½ cup dry quinoa - 1 cup water
- ½ cup diced cucumber
- ¼ cup cherry tomatoes, halved
- ¼ cup diced red onion
- 2 tablespoons lemon vinaigrette
- 1 teaspoon olive oil - ¼ teaspoon black pepper - ¼ teaspoon salt

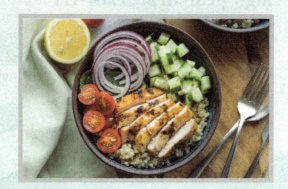

Instructions:

Rinse quinoa under cold water. - In a saucepan, bring quinoa and water to a boil. Reduce heat, cover, and simmer for 12-15 minutes until quinoa is tender. - In a large bowl, combine cooked quinoa, cucumber, cherry tomatoes, and red onion. - Top with grilled chicken slices. - Drizzle with lemon vinaigrette and olive oil. - Serve warm.

Nutritional Information (per serving):

Calories: 390 | Protein: 42g | Carbohydrates: 34g | Dietary Fiber: 6g | Sugars: 3g | Fat: 12g (Total), 3g (Saturated) | Cholesterol: 85mg | Sodium: 420mg

---

baked stuffed bell peppers

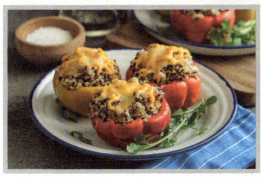

Ingredients (2 servings):

- 2 large bell peppers, halved and seeds removed
- 6 ounces lean ground turkey - ½ cup cooked quinoa
- ½ cup diced tomatoes - ¼ cup diced onions
- ½ teaspoon garlic powder - ½ teaspoon dried oregano
- ¼ teaspoon black pepper - ¼ teaspoon salt . ½ cup shredded low-fat cheddar cheese

Instructions:

Preheat oven to 375°F (190°C). - In a pan over medium heat, cook ground turkey until browned. - Stir in diced tomatoes, onions, garlic powder, oregano, salt, and pepper. - Mix in cooked quinoa and remove from heat. - Stuff each bell pepper half with the turkey-quinoa mixture. - Sprinkle with cheddar cheese. - Bake for 20 minutes until cheese is melted. - Serve warm.

Nutritional Information (per serving - 1 stuffed pepper):

Calories: 380 | Protein: 40g | Carbohydrates: 30g | Dietary Fiber: 7g | Sugars: 5g | Fat: 12g (Total), 4g (Saturated) | Cholesterol: 90mg | Sodium: 420mg

high-protein beef stir-fry

Ingredients (2 servings):

- 6 ounces lean beef, sliced thin
- 2 cups mixed stir-fry vegetables (bell peppers, broccoli, carrots)
- 1 teaspoon olive oil
- 1 tablespoon low-sodium soy sauce
- ½ teaspoon garlic powder
- ½ teaspoon ginger powder - ¼ teaspoon black pepper

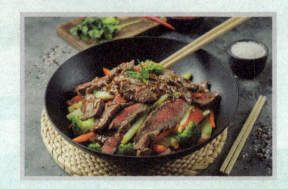

Instructions:

Heat olive oil in a large skillet over medium-high heat. - Add beef slices and cook for 2-3 minutes until browned. - Stir in mixed vegetables, soy sauce, garlic powder, ginger powder, and black pepper. - Stir-fry for another 3-4 minutes until vegetables are tender. - Serve warm.

Nutritional Information (per serving):

Calories: 420 | Protein: 45g | Carbohydrates: 14g | Dietary Fiber: 5g | Sugars: 6g | Fat: 14g (Total), 5g (Saturated) | Cholesterol: 95mg | Sodium: 430mg

---

salmon and asparagus foil pack

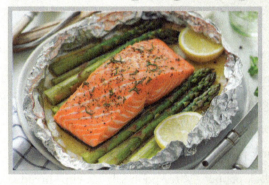

Ingredients (2 servings):

- 2 salmon fillets (6 oz each)
- 1 teaspoon olive oil
- ½ teaspoon lemon juice
- ½ teaspoon garlic powder
- ¼ teaspoon salt
- ¼ teaspoon black pepper
- 1 cup asparagus spears
- ¼ teaspoon dried thyme

Instructions:

Preheat oven to 375°F (190°C). - Place each salmon fillet on a sheet of foil. - Drizzle with olive oil and lemon juice. - Sprinkle with garlic powder, thyme, salt, and black pepper. - Arrange asparagus spears alongside the salmon. - Wrap the foil tightly to seal. - Bake for 15-18 minutes. - Serve warm.

Nutritional Information (per serving):

Calories: 390 | Protein: 42g | Carbohydrates: 4g | Dietary Fiber: 2g | Sugars: 1g | Fat: 20g (Total), 5g (Saturated) | Cholesterol: 90mg | Sodium: 330mg

shrimp and vegetable skewers

Ingredients (2 servings):
- 8 ounces shrimp, peeled and deveined
- ½ cup bell peppers, cut into chunks
- ½ cup zucchini, sliced
- ¼ cup red onion, cut into chunks
- 1 teaspoon olive oil
- ½ teaspoon garlic powder - ½ teaspoon paprika
- ¼ teaspoon black pepper - ¼ teaspoon salt - 2 wooden or metal skewers

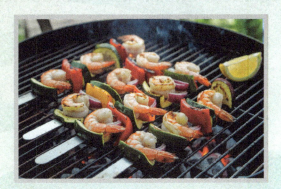

Instructions:

Preheat grill to medium-high heat. - In a bowl, toss shrimp and vegetables with olive oil, garlic powder, paprika, black pepper, and salt. - Thread shrimp and vegetables onto skewers. - Grill for 3-4 minutes per side until shrimp are opaque and vegetables are tender. - Serve immediately.

Nutritional Information (per serving):

Calories: 340 | Protein: 42g | Carbohydrates: 10g | Dietary Fiber: 3g | Sugars: 4g | Fat: 10g (Total), 2g (Saturated) | Cholesterol: 240mg | Sodium: 380mg

---

turkey and sweet potato skillet

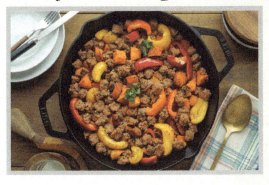

Ingredients (2 servings):
- 6 ounces lean ground turkey
- 1 medium sweet potato, peeled and diced
- ½ cup diced bell peppers
- ¼ cup diced onions
- 1 teaspoon olive oil - ½ teaspoon garlic powder
- ½ teaspoon smoked paprika - ¼ teaspoon black pepper - ¼ teaspoon salt

Instructions:

Heat olive oil in a large skillet over medium heat. - Add diced sweet potatoes and cook for 5 minutes, stirring occasionally. - Add onions and bell peppers, sauté for 3 more minutes. - Stir in ground turkey, garlic powder, smoked paprika, black pepper, and salt. - Cook for 6-8 minutes until turkey is fully cooked and sweet potatoes are tender. - Serve warm.

Nutritional Information (per serving):

Calories: 400 | Protein: 42g | Carbohydrates: 38g | Dietary Fiber: 6g | Sugars: 8g | Fat: 10g (Total), 2g (Saturated) | Cholesterol: 85mg | Sodium: 420mg

grilled chicken with avocado salsa

Ingredients (2 servings):
- 6 ounces grilled chicken breast
- ½ avocado, diced
- ¼ cup cherry tomatoes, halved
- ¼ cup diced red onion
- 1 teaspoon lime juice - ¼ teaspoon black pepper
- ¼ teaspoon salt - 1 teaspoon olive oil

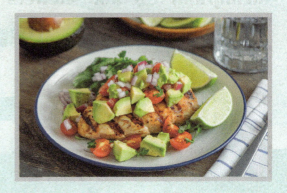

Instructions:

Season chicken with salt and black pepper, then grill over medium heat for 5-6 minutes per side. - In a bowl, mix avocado, cherry tomatoes, red onion, lime juice, and olive oil. - Spoon avocado salsa over grilled chicken and serve immediately.

Nutritional Information (per serving):

Calories: 380 | Protein: 44g | Carbohydrates: 10g | Dietary Fiber: 4g | Sugars: 3g | Fat: 14g (Total), 3g (Saturated) | Cholesterol: 90mg | Sodium: 380mg

---

zucchini noodles with turkey meatballs

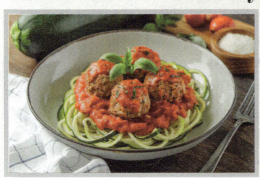

Ingredients (2 servings):
- 6 ounces lean ground turkey
- 1 zucchini, spiralized into noodles
- ¼ cup whole-wheat breadcrumbs
- 1 egg
- ½ teaspoon garlic powder
- ½ teaspoon dried oregano - ¼ teaspoon black pepper
- ¼ teaspoon salt - ½ cup marinara sauce - 1 teaspoon olive oil

Instructions:

Preheat oven to 375°F (190°C). - In a bowl, mix ground turkey, breadcrumbs, egg, garlic powder, oregano, black pepper, and salt. - Form into small meatballs and place on a baking sheet. - Bake for 15-18 minutes until cooked through. - Heat olive oil in a skillet over medium heat, sauté zucchini noodles for 2 minutes. - Add marinara sauce and cooked meatballs. - Serve warm.

Nutritional Information (per serving):

Calories: 360 | Protein: 42g | Carbohydrates: 22g | Dietary Fiber: 5g | Sugars: 6g | Fat: 12g (Total), 3g (Saturated) | Cholesterol: 110mg | Sodium: 450mg

spicy chicken & veggie bowl

Ingredients (2 servings):

- 6 ounces chicken breast, diced
- ½ cup cooked brown rice
- ½ cup steamed broccoli florets
- ¼ cup sliced bell peppers
- ¼ cup diced onions
- 1 teaspoon olive oil - ½ teaspoon chili powder
- ½ teaspoon garlic powder - ¼ teaspoon black pepper
- ¼ teaspoon salt

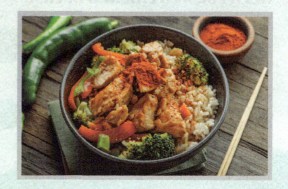

Instructions:

Heat olive oil in a skillet over medium heat. - Add chicken, chili powder, garlic powder, black pepper, and salt, cook for 5-6 minutes until browned. - Stir in bell peppers, onions, and steamed broccoli, sauté for 3 more minutes. - Serve over brown rice.

Nutritional Information (per serving):

Calories: 420 | Protein: 46g | Carbohydrates: 38g | Dietary Fiber: 6g | Sugars: 4g | Fat: 10g (Total), 2g (Saturated) | Cholesterol: 85mg | Sodium: 410mg

---

grilled tuna steaks

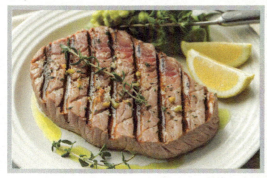

Ingredients (2 servings):

- 2 tuna steaks (6 oz each)
- 1 teaspoon olive oil
- ½ teaspoon lemon juice
- ½ teaspoon garlic powder
- ¼ teaspoon black pepper
- ¼ teaspoon salt
- ¼ teaspoon dried thyme

Instructions:

Preheat grill to medium-high heat. - Brush tuna steaks with olive oil and lemon juice. - Season with garlic powder, black pepper, salt, and thyme. - Grill for 3-4 minutes per side for medium-rare, or longer for well-done. - Serve immediately.

Nutritional Information (per serving):

Calories: 380 | Protein: 44g | Carbohydrates: 2g | Dietary Fiber: 0g | Sugars: 0g | Fat: 18g (Total), 4g (Saturated) | Cholesterol: 80mg | Sodium: 330mg

herb roasted chicken breast

Ingredients (2 servings):

- 2 boneless, skinless chicken breasts (6 oz each)
- 1 teaspoon olive oil
- ½ teaspoon garlic powder
- ½ teaspoon dried rosemary
- ½ teaspoon dried thyme
- ¼ teaspoon salt - ¼ teaspoon black pepper

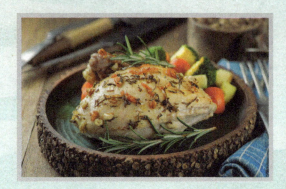

Instructions:

Preheat oven to 375°F (190°C). - Rub chicken breasts with olive oil. - Mix garlic powder, rosemary, thyme, salt, and black pepper, then coat the chicken with the mixture. - Place on a baking sheet and bake for 20-25 minutes until fully cooked. - Let rest for 5 minutes before serving.

Nutritional Information (per serving):

Calories: 340 | Protein: 42g | Carbohydrates: 2g | Dietary Fiber: 0g | Sugars: 0g | Fat: 14g (Total), 3g (Saturated) | Cholesterol: 110mg | Sodium: 350mg

---

beef and broccoli protein bowl

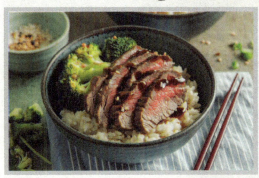

Ingredients (2 servings):

- 6 ounces lean beef, sliced thin
- 2 cups broccoli florets
- ½ cup cooked brown rice
- 1 teaspoon olive oil
- 1 tablespoon low-sodium soy sauce
- ½ teaspoon garlic powder - ¼ teaspoon black pepper
- ¼ teaspoon ginger powder

Instructions:

Heat olive oil in a large skillet over medium-high heat. - Add beef slices and cook for 3-4 minutes until browned. - Stir in broccoli florets, soy sauce, garlic powder, black pepper, and ginger powder. - Cook for another 4 minutes until broccoli is tender. - Serve over brown rice.

Nutritional Information (per serving):

Calories: 420 | Protein: 44g | Carbohydrates: 36g | Dietary Fiber: 6g | Sugars: 4g | Fat: 12g (Total), 4g (Saturated) | Cholesterol: 85mg | Sodium: 450mg

chicken cauliflower fried rice

Ingredients (2 servings):
- 6 ounces chicken breast, diced
- 2 cups riced cauliflower
- ½ cup diced carrots - ¼ cup diced onions
- ½ teaspoon garlic powder
- ½ teaspoon low-sodium soy sauce
- 1 teaspoon olive oil
- ¼ teaspoon black pepper - 1 egg, scrambled

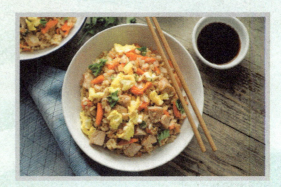

Instructions:

Heat olive oil in a large skillet over medium heat. - Add diced chicken and cook for 5-6 minutes until browned. - Stir in carrots, onions, garlic powder, and black pepper. - Add riced cauliflower and soy sauce, cook for another 3 minutes. - Stir in scrambled egg and mix well. - Serve hot.

Nutritional Information (per serving):

Calories: 380 | Protein: 42g | Carbohydrates: 16g | Dietary Fiber: 5g | Sugars: 5g | Fat: 14g (Total), 3g (Saturated) | Cholesterol: 220mg | Sodium: 400mg

---

baked tilapia with veggies

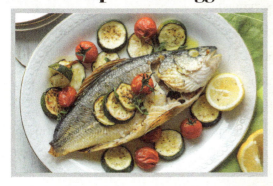

Ingredients (2 servings):
- 2 tilapia fillets (6 oz each)
- 1 teaspoon olive oil
- ½ teaspoon lemon juice
- ½ teaspoon garlic powder
- ¼ teaspoon black pepper
- ¼ teaspoon salt - ½ cup sliced zucchini
- ½ cup cherry tomatoes, halved

Instructions:

Preheat oven to 375°F (190°C). - Place tilapia fillets on a baking sheet lined with parchment paper. - Drizzle with olive oil and lemon juice. - Season with garlic powder, black pepper, and salt. - Arrange zucchini and cherry tomatoes around the fillets. - Bake for 12-15 minutes until fish is flaky. - Serve warm.

Nutritional Information (per serving):

Calories: 320 | Protein: 40g | Carbohydrates: 8g | Dietary Fiber: 2g | Sugars: 3g | Fat: 12g (Total), 3g (Saturated) | Cholesterol: 75mg | Sodium: 340mg

high-protein taco salad

Ingredients (2 servings):

- 6 ounces lean ground turkey
- 4 cups chopped romaine lettuce
- ½ cup diced tomatoes - ¼ cup diced red onion
- ¼ cup shredded low-fat cheddar cheese
- 2 tablespoons Greek yogurt (for dressing)
- ½ teaspoon taco seasoning - ¼ teaspoon black pepper - 1 teaspoon olive oil

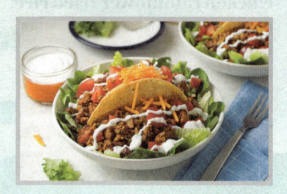

Instructions:

Heat olive oil in a skillet over medium heat. - Add ground turkey and taco seasoning, cook for 5-6 minutes until browned. - In two serving bowls, divide romaine lettuce evenly. - Top with cooked turkey, diced tomatoes, red onion, and shredded cheddar cheese. - Drizzle with Greek yogurt and serve immediately.

Nutritional Information (per serving):

Calories: 400 | Protein: 42g | Carbohydrates: 14g | Dietary Fiber: 5g | Sugars: 3g | Fat: 16g (Total), 4g (Saturated) | Cholesterol: 85mg | Sodium: 420mg

---

spaghetti squash with turkey bolognese

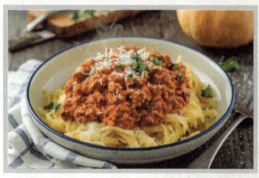

Ingredients (2 servings):

- 1 medium spaghetti squash - 6 ounces lean ground turkey
- ½ cup marinara sauce (low-sodium)
- ¼ cup diced onions - ½ teaspoon garlic powder
- ½ teaspoon dried oregano - ¼ teaspoon black pepper
- ¼ teaspoon salt - ½ teaspoon olive oil - ¼ cup grated Parmesan cheese

Instructions:

Preheat oven to 375°F (190°C). - Cut the spaghetti squash in half lengthwise and remove seeds. - Drizzle the inside with olive oil and season with salt and pepper. - Place cut-side down on a baking sheet and bake for 35-40 minutes, or until fork-tender. - Meanwhile, heat a pan over medium heat and cook ground turkey until browned. - Stir in diced onions, marinara sauce, garlic powder, and oregano. - Simmer for 5-7 minutes until sauce thickens. - Once the squash is done, use a fork to scrape out spaghetti-like strands. - Top with turkey Bolognese and sprinkle with Parmesan cheese. - Serve warm.

Nutritional Information (per serving):

Calories: 400 | Protein: 42g | Carbohydrates: 28g | Dietary Fiber: 6g | Sugars: 8g | Fat: 12g (Total), 4g (Saturated) | Cholesterol: 85mg | Sodium: 420mg

chicken parmesan (low-carb)

Ingredients (2 servings):
- 2 boneless, skinless chicken breasts (6 oz each)
- ½ cup marinara sauce
- ½ cup shredded low-fat mozzarella cheese
- ¼ cup grated Parmesan cheese
- ½ teaspoon garlic powder
- ½ teaspoon dried oregano - ¼ teaspoon black pepper
- ¼ teaspoon salt - 1 teaspoon olive oil

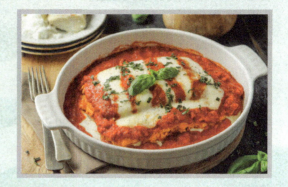

Instructions:

Preheat oven to 375°F (190°C). - Heat olive oil in a skillet over medium heat and cook chicken breasts for 3-4 minutes per side until golden. - Place chicken in a baking dish and top with marinara sauce, mozzarella, Parmesan, garlic powder, oregano, black pepper, and salt. - Bake for 15 minutes until cheese is bubbly. - Serve warm.

Nutritional Information (per serving):

Calories: 400 | Protein: 48g | Carbohydrates: 10g | Dietary Fiber: 2g | Sugars: 5g | Fat: 14g (Total), 6g (Saturated) | Cholesterol: 110mg | Sodium: 420mg

---

spicy shrimp stir-fry

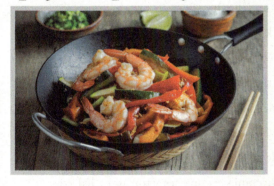

Ingredients (2 servings):
- 8 ounces shrimp, peeled and deveined
- ½ cup sliced bell peppers
- ½ cup zucchini, sliced
- ¼ cup diced onions
- 1 teaspoon olive oil - 1 teaspoon low-sodium soy sauce
- ½ teaspoon red pepper flakes - ¼ teaspoon garlic powder - ¼ teaspoon black pepper

Instructions:

Heat olive oil in a skillet over medium heat. - Add onions, bell peppers, and zucchini, sauté for 3 minutes. - Stir in shrimp, soy sauce, red pepper flakes, garlic powder, and black pepper. - Cook for another 3-4 minutes until shrimp turn pink and opaque. - Serve immediately.

Nutritional Information (per serving):

Calories: 320 | Protein: 42g | Carbohydrates: 12g | Dietary Fiber: 4g | Sugars: 3g | Fat: 10g (Total), 2g (Saturated) | Cholesterol: 240mg | Sodium: 380mg

italian meatball bake

Ingredients (2 servings):

- 6 ounces lean ground turkey
- ¼ cup whole-wheat breadcrumbs
- 1 egg
- ½ teaspoon garlic powder - ½ teaspoon dried basil
- ¼ teaspoon black pepper - ¼ teaspoon salt
- ½ cup marinara sauce - ½ cup shredded mozzarella cheese - 1 teaspoon olive oil

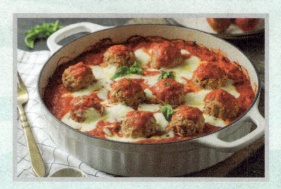

Instructions:

Preheat oven to 375°F (190°C). - In a bowl, mix ground turkey, breadcrumbs, egg, garlic powder, basil, black pepper, and salt. - Form into small meatballs and place in a greased baking dish. - Pour marinara sauce over meatballs and top with mozzarella cheese. - Bake for 20-25 minutes until cheese is bubbly. - Serve warm.

Nutritional Information (per serving):

Calories: 380 | Protein: 42g | Carbohydrates: 14g | Dietary Fiber: 3g | Sugars: 5g | Fat: 14g (Total), 5g (Saturated) | Cholesterol: 110mg | Sodium: 450mg

---

grilled pork chops with veggies

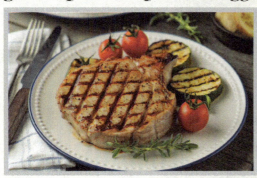

Ingredients (2 servings):

- 2 boneless pork chops (6 oz each)
- 1 teaspoon olive oil
- ½ teaspoon garlic powder
- ½ teaspoon dried rosemary
- ¼ teaspoon black pepper
- ¼ teaspoon salt
- ½ cup sliced zucchini - ½ cup cherry tomatoes, halved

Instructions:

Preheat grill to medium-high heat. - Rub pork chops with olive oil, garlic powder, rosemary, black pepper, and salt. - Grill for 5-6 minutes per side until fully cooked. - Grill zucchini and cherry tomatoes for 3-4 minutes until tender. - Serve pork chops with grilled vegetables.

Nutritional Information (per serving):

Calories: 420 | Protein: 48g | Carbohydrates: 10g | Dietary Fiber: 3g | Sugars: 4g | Fat: 18g (Total), 6g (Saturated) | Cholesterol: 110mg | Sodium: 400mg

HIGH PROTEIN COOKBOOK

teriyaki chicken protein bowl

Ingredients (2 servings):
- 6 ounces chicken breast, diced
- ½ cup cooked brown rice
- ½ cup steamed broccoli florets
- ¼ cup sliced bell peppers
- ¼ cup shredded carrots
- 1 teaspoon olive oil
- 1 tablespoon low-sodium teriyaki sauce
- ¼ teaspoon garlic powder - ¼ teaspoon black pepper

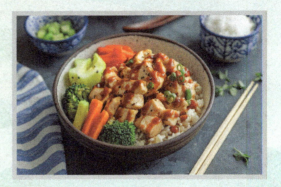

Instructions:

Heat olive oil in a skillet over medium heat. - Add diced chicken and cook for 5-6 minutes until browned. - Stir in bell peppers, carrots, and broccoli, sauté for 3 minutes. - Add teriyaki sauce, garlic powder, and black pepper, toss to coat evenly. - Serve over brown rice.

Nutritional Information (per serving):

Calories: 420 | Protein: 45g | Carbohydrates: 36g | Dietary Fiber: 6g | Sugars: 5g | Fat: 10g (Total), 2g (Saturated) | Cholesterol: 90mg | Sodium: 420mg

---

lemon garlic chicken breasts

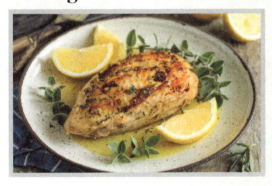

Ingredients (2 servings):
- 2 boneless, skinless chicken breasts (6 oz each)
- 1 teaspoon olive oil
- ½ teaspoon lemon juice
- ½ teaspoon garlic powder
- ¼ teaspoon black pepper
- ¼ teaspoon salt
- ½ teaspoon dried oregano

Instructions:

Preheat oven to 375°F (190°C). - Rub chicken breasts with olive oil and lemon juice. - Season with garlic powder, oregano, black pepper, and salt. - Bake for 20-25 minutes until fully cooked. - Let rest for 5 minutes before serving.

Nutritional Information (per serving):

Calories: 340 | Protein: 42g | Carbohydrates: 2g | Dietary Fiber: 0g | Sugars: 0g | Fat: 14g (Total), 3g (Saturated) | Cholesterol: 110mg | Sodium: 350mg

turkey zucchini burgers

Ingredients (2 servings):
- 6 ounces lean ground turkey
- ½ cup grated zucchini
- ¼ cup whole-wheat breadcrumbs
- 1 egg
- ½ teaspoon garlic powder
- ¼ teaspoon black pepper - ¼ teaspoon salt
- 1 teaspoon olive oil

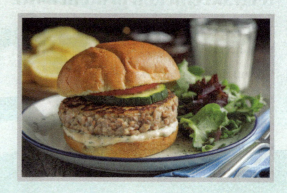

Instructions:

In a bowl, mix ground turkey, grated zucchini, breadcrumbs, egg, garlic powder, black pepper, and salt. - Form into two patties. - Heat olive oil in a skillet over medium heat. - Cook patties for 4-5 minutes per side until fully cooked. - Serve with a side of mixed greens.

Nutritional Information (per serving - 1 burger):

Calories: 360 | Protein: 40g | Carbohydrates: 12g | Dietary Fiber: 3g | Sugars: 2g | Fat: 14g (Total), 4g (Saturated) | Cholesterol: 110mg | Sodium: 380mg

---

baked salmon with dill sauce

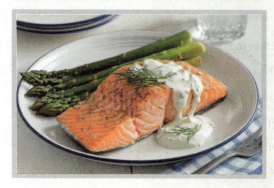

Ingredients (2 servings):
- 2 salmon fillets (6 oz each)
- 1 teaspoon olive oil
- ½ teaspoon garlic powder
- ¼ teaspoon salt
- ¼ teaspoon black pepper
- ½ cup Greek yogurt (plain, non-fat)
- 1 teaspoon fresh dill, chopped - ½ teaspoon lemon juice

Instructions:

Preheat oven to 375°F (190°C). - Place salmon fillets on a baking sheet lined with parchment paper. - Drizzle with olive oil and season with garlic powder, salt, and black pepper. - Bake for 12-15 minutes until flaky. - In a small bowl, mix Greek yogurt, dill, and lemon juice. - Serve salmon topped with dill sauce.

Nutritional Information (per serving):

Calories: 400 | Protein: 44g | Carbohydrates: 4g | Dietary Fiber: 0g | Sugars: 2g | Fat: 20g (Total), 5g (Saturated) | Cholesterol: 85mg | Sodium: 340mg

protein veggie lasagna

Ingredients (2 servings):

- 4 whole-wheat lasagna noodles
- 6 ounces lean ground turkey
- ½ cup low-fat ricotta cheese
- ½ cup marinara sauce - ½ cup diced zucchini
- ¼ cup diced mushrooms - ¼ teaspoon garlic powder
- ¼ teaspoon black pepper - ½ teaspoon dried basil - ½ cup shredded low-fat mozzarella cheese

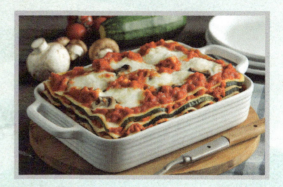

Instructions:

Preheat oven to 375°F (190°C). - Cook lasagna noodles according to package instructions. - Heat a skillet over medium heat and cook ground turkey until browned. - Stir in diced zucchini, mushrooms, garlic powder, black pepper, and marinara sauce, then remove from heat. - In a baking dish, layer cooked noodles, ricotta cheese, turkey mixture, and shredded mozzarella. - Repeat layers and top with remaining cheese. - Bake for 25 minutes until bubbly. - Serve warm.

Nutritional Information (per serving):

Calories: 450 | Protein: 48g | Carbohydrates: 42g | Dietary Fiber: 8g | Sugars: 6g | Fat: 12g (Total), 5g (Saturated) | Cholesterol: 90mg | Sodium: 450mg

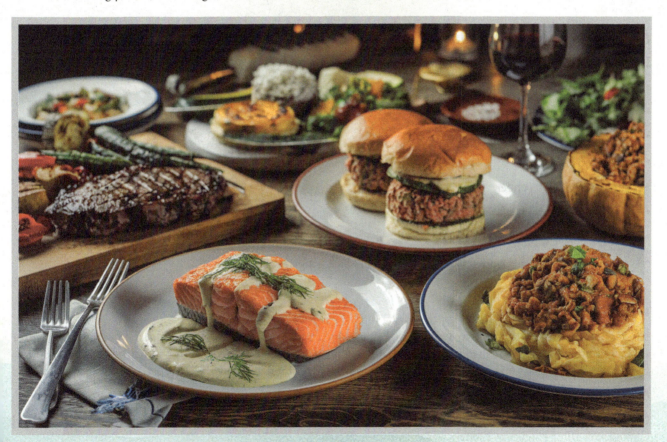

main vegetarian recipes

・・・

High Protein, Plant-Based Options

Eating plant-based doesn't mean sacrificing protein! These vegetarian and vegan recipes are rich in plant-based protein sources like lentils, chickpeas, tofu, quinoa, and black beans. They are designed to provide essential nutrients while keeping you full and energized. Each meal is packed with flavor, easy to prepare, and perfect for a high-protein diet.

chickpea & quinoa salad

Ingredients (2 servings):

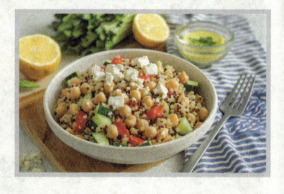

- ½ cup dry quinoa
- 1 cup water
- ½ cup canned chickpeas, drained and rinsed
- ½ cup diced cucumber
- ¼ cup diced red bell pepper
- ¼ cup crumbled feta cheese (optional)
- 2 tablespoons lemon juice
- 1 teaspoon olive oil - ½ teaspoon cumin - ¼ teaspoon black pepper - ¼ teaspoon salt

Instructions:

Rinse quinoa under cold water. - In a saucepan, bring quinoa and water to a boil. Reduce heat, cover, and simmer for 12-15 minutes until quinoa is tender. - In a large bowl, mix quinoa, chickpeas, cucumber, red bell pepper, and feta cheese. - Drizzle with lemon juice and olive oil, then season with cumin, salt, and black pepper. - Toss well and serve.

Nutritional Information (per serving):

Calories: 320 | Protein: 18g | Carbohydrates: 40g | Dietary Fiber: 8g | Sugars: 4g | Fat: 10g (Total), 2g (Saturated) | Cholesterol: 10mg | Sodium: 320mg

tofu & veggie stir-fry

Ingredients (2 servings):
- 6 ounces firm tofu, cubed
- 2 cups mixed stir-fry vegetables (bell peppers, carrots, broccoli)
- 1 teaspoon olive oil
- 1 tablespoon low-sodium soy sauce
- ½ teaspoon garlic powder
- ½ teaspoon ginger powder
- ¼ teaspoon black pepper

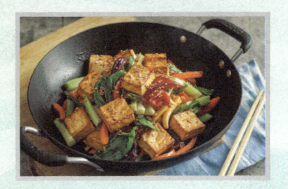

Instructions:
Heat olive oil in a large skillet over medium-high heat. - Add tofu cubes and cook for 3-4 minutes until golden brown. - Stir in mixed vegetables, soy sauce, garlic powder, ginger powder, and black pepper. - Stir-fry for another 4 minutes until vegetables are tender. - Serve warm.

Nutritional Information (per serving):

Calories: 340 | Protein: 30g | Carbohydrates: 22g | Dietary Fiber: 6g | Sugars: 4g | Fat: 14g (Total), 2g (Saturated) | Cholesterol: 0mg | Sodium: 400mg

---

high-protein lentil curry

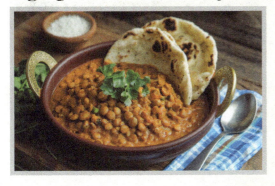

Ingredients (2 servings):
- ½ cup dry lentils, rinsed
- 2 cups low-sodium vegetable broth
- ½ cup diced tomatoes
- ¼ cup diced onion
- ½ teaspoon garlic powder
- ½ teaspoon curry powder - ¼ teaspoon black pepper
- ¼ teaspoon salt - 1 teaspoon olive oil

Instructions:
Heat olive oil in a pot over medium heat. - Add onions and sauté for 2 minutes. - Stir in lentils, diced tomatoes, curry powder, garlic powder, black pepper, and salt. - Add vegetable broth and bring to a boil. - Reduce heat and simmer for 25-30 minutes until lentils are tender. - Serve warm.

Nutritional Information (per serving):

Calories: 360 | Protein: 22g | Carbohydrates: 40g | Dietary Fiber: 10g | Sugars: 5g | Fat: 8g (Total), 1g (Saturated) | Cholesterol: 0mg | Sodium: 350mg

black bean veggie burger

Ingredients (2 servings):

- 1 cup canned black beans, drained and rinsed
- ¼ cup whole-wheat breadcrumbs
- ¼ cup diced onions
- ½ teaspoon garlic powder
- ½ teaspoon smoked paprika
- ¼ teaspoon black pepper - ¼ teaspoon salt - 1 teaspoon olive oil

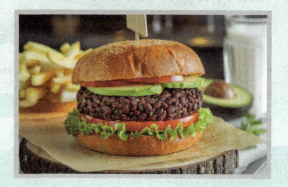

Instructions:

Mash black beans in a bowl until mostly smooth. - Stir in breadcrumbs, onions, garlic powder, smoked paprika, black pepper, and salt. - Form into two patties. - Heat olive oil in a skillet over medium heat. - Cook patties for 4-5 minutes per side until firm and golden brown. - Serve with whole-wheat buns or lettuce wraps.

Nutritional Information (per serving - 1 burger):

Calories: 320 | Protein: 22g | Carbohydrates: 36g | Dietary Fiber: 10g | Sugars: 2g | Fat: 8g (Total), 1g (Saturated) | Cholesterol: 0mg | Sodium: 350mg

---

crispy tofu & edamame stir-fry

Ingredients (2 servings):

- 6 ounces firm tofu, cubed - ½ cup shelled edamame
- ½ cup sliced bell peppers - ¼ cup sliced carrots
- ¼ cup diced onions - 1 teaspoon olive oil
- 1 tablespoon low-sodium soy sauce - ½ teaspoon garlic powder
- ½ teaspoon ginger powder - ¼ teaspoon black pepper - ¼ teaspoon red pepper flakes (optional)

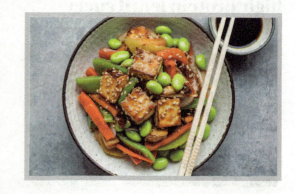

Instructions:

Pat tofu dry and cut into cubes. - Heat olive oil in a skillet over medium-high heat. - Add tofu cubes and cook for 5 minutes, turning occasionally, until crispy. - Remove tofu from the skillet and set aside. - In the same skillet, add onions, bell peppers, and carrots, sauté for 3 minutes. - Stir in edamame, soy sauce, garlic powder, ginger powder, black pepper, and red pepper flakes. - Return tofu to the pan and toss everything together for another 2 minutes. - Serve immediately.

Nutritional Information (per serving):

Calories: 380 | Protein: 34g | Carbohydrates: 26g | Dietary Fiber: 8g | Sugars: 5g | Fat: 14g (Total), 2g (Saturated) | Cholesterol: 0mg | Sodium: 400mg

spicy bean chili

Ingredients (2 servings):

- ½ cup canned black beans, drained and rinsed
- ½ cup canned kidney beans, drained and rinsed
- 1 cup diced tomatoes
- ½ cup diced bell peppers
- ¼ cup diced onions
- 1 teaspoon olive oil - ½ teaspoon chili powder
- ½ teaspoon cumin - ¼ teaspoon garlic powder - ¼ teaspoon salt - ½ cup low-sodium vegetable broth

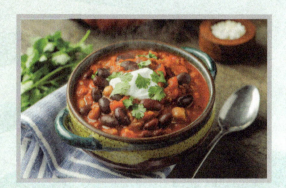

Instructions:

Heat olive oil in a pot over medium heat. - Add onions and bell peppers, sauté for 3 minutes. - Stir in black beans, kidney beans, diced tomatoes, chili powder, cumin, garlic powder, salt, and vegetable broth. - Bring to a boil, then reduce heat and let simmer for 20 minutes. - Serve warm.

Nutritional Information (per serving):

Calories: 380 | Protein: 22g | Carbohydrates: 42g | Dietary Fiber: 12g | Sugars: 6g | Fat: 8g (Total), 1g (Saturated) | Cholesterol: 0mg | Sodium: 380mg

---

protein pasta with spinach and chickpeas

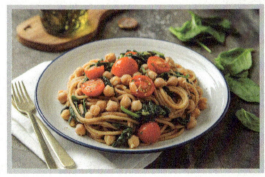

Ingredients (2 servings):

- 4 ounces whole-wheat pasta
- ½ cup canned chickpeas, drained and rinsed
- 1 cup baby spinach
- ¼ cup diced cherry tomatoes - 1 teaspoon olive oil
- ½ teaspoon garlic powder - ¼ teaspoon black pepper
- ¼ teaspoon salt - ¼ teaspoon red pepper flakes

Instructions:

Cook whole-wheat pasta according to package instructions. - Heat olive oil in a pan over medium heat. - Add chickpeas, garlic powder, black pepper, salt, and red pepper flakes, sauté for 3 minutes. - Stir in spinach and cherry tomatoes, cook for another 2 minutes. - Mix with cooked pasta and serve warm.

Nutritional Information (per serving):

Calories: 390 | Protein: 22g | Carbohydrates: 48g | Dietary Fiber: 8g | Sugars: 5g | Fat: 10g (Total), 2g (Saturated) | Cholesterol: 0mg | Sodium: 360mg

vegan buddha bowl

Ingredients (2 servings):

- ½ cup cooked quinoa
- ½ cup canned black beans, drained and rinsed
- ½ cup roasted sweet potatoes, diced
- ½ cup steamed broccoli
- ¼ avocado, sliced
- 2 tablespoons tahini dressing
- ¼ teaspoon black pepper - ¼ teaspoon salt

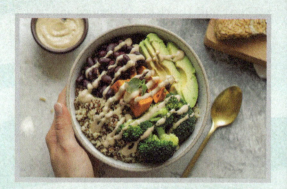

Instructions:

Divide cooked quinoa between two bowls. - Top with black beans, roasted sweet potatoes, steamed broccoli, and avocado slices. - Drizzle with tahini dressing. - Sprinkle with salt and black pepper. - Serve immediately.

Nutritional Information (per serving):

Calories: 420 | Protein: 22g | Carbohydrates: 42g | Dietary Fiber: 10g | Sugars: 5g | Fat: 14g (Total), 3g (Saturated) | Cholesterol: 0mg | Sodium: 340mg

mushroom & lentil tacos

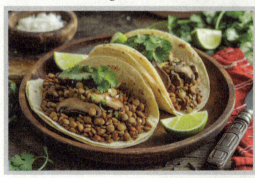

Ingredients (2 servings):

- ½ cup cooked lentils
- ½ cup sliced mushrooms
- ¼ cup diced onions
- 1 teaspoon olive oil - ½ teaspoon cumin
- ¼ teaspoon garlic powder - ¼ teaspoon black pepper
- ¼ teaspoon salt - 4 small corn tortillas

Instructions:

Heat olive oil in a skillet over medium heat. - Add onions and mushrooms, sauté for 3 minutes. - Stir in cooked lentils, cumin, garlic powder, black pepper, and salt, cook for another 3 minutes. - Warm corn tortillas and fill with lentil-mushroom mixture. - Serve warm.

Nutritional Information (per serving - 2 tacos):

Calories: 350 | Protein: 20g | Carbohydrates: 42g | Dietary Fiber: 8g | Sugars: 3g | Fat: 8g (Total), 1g (Saturated) | Cholesterol: 0mg | Sodium: 320mg

HIGH PROTEIN COOKBOOK

high protein falafel wrap

Ingredients (2 servings):

- ½ cup canned chickpeas, drained and rinsed
- ¼ cup whole-wheat breadcrumbs
- ¼ teaspoon cumin
- ¼ teaspoon garlic powder
- ¼ teaspoon black pepper
- ¼ teaspoon salt - 1 teaspoon olive oil
- 2 whole-wheat tortillas - ½ cup shredded lettuce - ¼ cup diced tomatoes - 2 tablespoons hummus

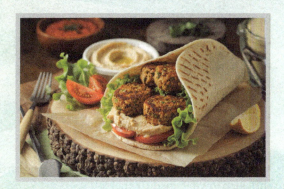

Instructions:

Mash chickpeas in a bowl until slightly chunky. - Stir in breadcrumbs, cumin, garlic powder, black pepper, and salt. - Form into small patties. - Heat olive oil in a skillet over medium heat and cook patties for 3 minutes per side until golden brown. - Spread hummus on tortillas, add lettuce, tomatoes, and falafel patties. - Wrap tightly and serve.

Nutritional Information (per serving - 1 wrap):

Calories: 380 | Protein: 22g | Carbohydrates: 42g | Dietary Fiber: 9g | Sugars: 4g | Fat: 10g (Total), 2g (Saturated) | Cholesterol: 0mg | Sodium: 360mg

---

chickpea salad sandwich

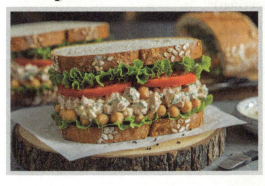

Ingredients (2 servings):

- 1 cup canned chickpeas, drained and rinsed
- ¼ cup Greek yogurt (plain, non-fat)
- ¼ teaspoon Dijon mustard
- ¼ teaspoon garlic powder
- ¼ teaspoon black pepper - ¼ teaspoon salt
- ¼ cup diced celery - 4 slices whole-wheat bread - 2 lettuce leaves - 2 tomato slices

Instructions:

Mash chickpeas in a bowl until slightly chunky. - Stir in Greek yogurt, Dijon mustard, garlic powder, black pepper, salt, and diced celery. - Spread the mixture evenly over two slices of whole-wheat bread. - Top with lettuce and tomato slices, then cover with the remaining bread slices. - Serve immediately.

Nutritional Information (per serving - 1 sandwich):

Calories: 380 | Protein: 22g | Carbohydrates: 45g | Dietary Fiber: 9g | Sugars: 5g | Fat: 8g (Total), 2g (Saturated) | Cholesterol: 5mg | Sodium: 360mg

black bean enchiladas

Ingredients (2 servings):

- 1 cup canned black beans, drained and rinsed
- ¼ cup diced onions
- ¼ cup diced bell peppers
- ½ teaspoon cumin - ¼ teaspoon garlic powder
- ¼ teaspoon black pepper - ¼ teaspoon salt
- ½ cup enchilada sauce - 2 whole-wheat tortillas - ¼ cup shredded low-fat cheddar cheese

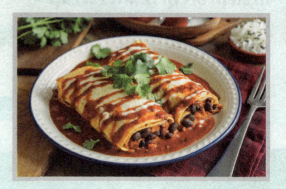

Instructions:

Preheat oven to 375°F (190°C). - In a pan over medium heat, sauté onions and bell peppers for 3 minutes. - Stir in black beans, cumin, garlic powder, black pepper, and salt, cook for another 3 minutes. - Divide the mixture between tortillas, roll them up, and place in a baking dish. - Pour enchilada sauce over the top and sprinkle with cheese. - Bake for 15-20 minutes until cheese is melted. - Serve warm.

Nutritional Information (per serving - 1 enchilada):

Calories: 400 | Protein: 24g | Carbohydrates: 46g | Dietary Fiber: 10g | Sugars: 6g | Fat: 10g (Total), 3g (Saturated) | Cholesterol: 15mg | Sodium: 420mg

---

vegetarian eggplant parmesan

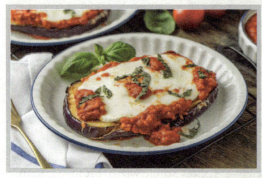

Ingredients (2 servings):

- 1 medium eggplant, sliced into rounds
- ½ cup whole-wheat breadcrumbs
- ¼ cup grated Parmesan cheese - ½ teaspoon garlic powder
- ¼ teaspoon black pepper - ¼ teaspoon salt
- 1 egg, beaten - ½ cup marinara sauce - ¼ cup shredded low-fat mozzarella cheese - 1 teaspoon olive oil

Instructions:

Preheat oven to 375°F (190°C). - In a shallow bowl, mix breadcrumbs, Parmesan cheese, garlic powder, black pepper, and salt. - Dip each eggplant slice into the beaten egg, then coat with the breadcrumb mixture. - Heat olive oil in a skillet over medium heat and cook eggplant slices for 2-3 minutes per side until golden brown. - Transfer to a baking dish, top with marinara sauce and mozzarella cheese. - Bake for 15 minutes until cheese is melted. - Serve warm.

Nutritional Information (per serving):

Calories: 380 | Protein: 24g | Carbohydrates: 36g | Dietary Fiber: 8g | Sugars: 6g | Fat: 12g (Total), 4g (Saturated) | Cholesterol: 75mg | Sodium: 400mg

quinoa and veggie protein bowl

Ingredients (2 servings):

- ½ cup cooked quinoa
- ½ cup roasted chickpeas
- ½ cup steamed kale
- ¼ cup diced bell peppers
- ¼ cup shredded carrots
- 2 tablespoons tahini dressing
- ¼ teaspoon black pepper - ¼ teaspoon salt

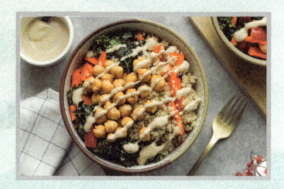

Instructions:

Divide cooked quinoa between two bowls. - Top with roasted chickpeas, steamed kale, diced bell peppers, and shredded carrots. - Drizzle with tahini dressing. - Sprinkle with black pepper and salt. - Serve immediately.

Nutritional Information (per serving):

Calories: 420 | Protein: 22g | Carbohydrates: 42g | Dietary Fiber: 10g | Sugars: 5g | Fat: 14g (Total), 3g (Saturated) | Cholesterol: 0mg | Sodium: 340mg

---

lentil and mushroom burgers

Ingredients (2 servings):

- ½ cup cooked lentils
- ½ cup diced mushrooms
- ¼ cup whole-wheat breadcrumbs
- 1 egg
- ½ teaspoon garlic powder
- ¼ teaspoon black pepper
- ¼ teaspoon salt
- 1 teaspoon olive oil

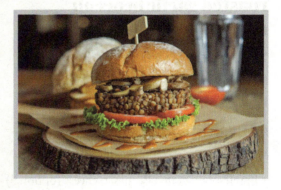

Instructions:

Mash cooked lentils in a bowl until slightly chunky. - Stir in diced mushrooms, breadcrumbs, egg, garlic powder, black pepper, and salt. - Form into two patties. - Heat olive oil in a skillet over medium heat. - Cook patties for 4-5 minutes per side until firm and golden brown. - Serve on whole-wheat buns or lettuce wraps.

Nutritional Information (per serving - 1 burger):

Calories: 350 | Protein: 24g | Carbohydrates: 40g | Dietary Fiber: 9g | Sugars: 4g | Fat: 8g (Total), 2g (Saturated) | Cholesterol: 55mg | Sodium: 350mg

sides recipes

...

Nutritious Complements to Any Meal

Side dishes are an essential part of a balanced diet, providing extra nutrients, flavors, and textures to complement any meal. These high-protein side dishes are not only nutritious but also quick and easy to prepare. Whether you need a refreshing salad, a crispy vegetable dish, or a warm roasted side, these recipes will enhance your meals while keeping them light and wholesome.

roasted garlic broccoli

Ingredients (2 servings):

- 2 cups broccoli florets
- 1 teaspoon olive oil
- 2 cloves garlic, minced
- ¼ teaspoon black pepper
- ¼ teaspoon salt
- 1 tablespoon grated Parmesan cheese (optional)

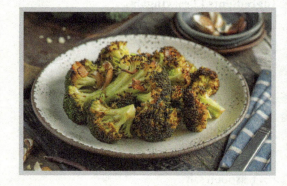

Instructions:

Preheat oven to 400°F (200°C). - In a bowl, toss broccoli florets with olive oil, minced garlic, black pepper, and salt. - Spread evenly on a baking sheet lined with parchment paper. - Roast for 15-20 minutes until tender and slightly crispy. - Sprinkle with Parmesan cheese if desired. - Serve warm.

Nutritional Information (per serving):

Calories: 140 | Protein: 8g | Carbohydrates: 12g | Dietary Fiber: 5g | Sugars: 3g | Fat: 6g (Total), 1g (Saturated) | Cholesterol: 5mg | Sodium: 180mg

quinoa salad

Ingredients (2 servings):

- ½ cup dry quinoa
- 1 cup water
- ¼ cup diced cucumbers
- ¼ cup diced bell peppers
- ¼ cup cherry tomatoes, halved
- 1 tablespoon lemon juice
- 1 teaspoon olive oil - ¼ teaspoon black pepper - ¼ teaspoon salt

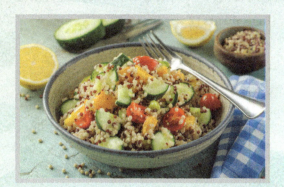

Instructions:

Rinse quinoa under cold water. - In a saucepan, bring quinoa and water to a boil. Reduce heat, cover, and simmer for 12-15 minutes until quinoa is tender. - In a large bowl, mix quinoa, cucumbers, bell peppers, and cherry tomatoes. - Drizzle with lemon juice and olive oil, then season with black pepper and salt. - Toss well and serve chilled or at room temperature.

Nutritional Information (per serving):

Calories: 180 | Protein: 7g | Carbohydrates: 30g | Dietary Fiber: 5g | Sugars: 4g | Fat: 5g (Total), 1g (Saturated) | Cholesterol: 0mg | Sodium: 150mg

---

cauliflower rice

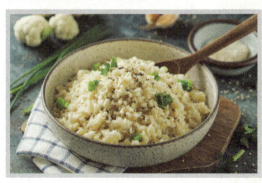

Ingredients (2 servings):

- 2 cups cauliflower, grated into rice-like pieces
- 1 teaspoon olive oil
- ½ teaspoon garlic powder
- ¼ teaspoon black pepper
- ¼ teaspoon salt

Instructions:

Heat olive oil in a skillet over medium heat. - Add grated cauliflower and cook for 3-4 minutes, stirring occasionally. - Stir in garlic powder, black pepper, and salt. - Cook for another 2 minutes until cauliflower is tender but not mushy. - Serve warm.

Nutritional Information (per serving):

Calories: 80 | Protein: 5g | Carbohydrates: 10g | Dietary Fiber: 3g | Sugars: 3g | Fat: 3g (Total), 0g (Saturated) | Cholesterol: 0mg | Sodium: 140mg

grilled asparagus with lemon

Ingredients (2 servings):

- 1 bunch asparagus, trimmed
- 1 teaspoon olive oil
- ½ teaspoon lemon juice
- ¼ teaspoon black pepper
- ¼ teaspoon salt

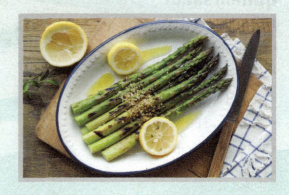

Instructions:

Preheat grill to medium heat. - In a bowl, toss asparagus with olive oil, lemon juice, black pepper, and salt. - Place asparagus spears on the grill and cook for 3-4 minutes per side until tender. - Serve warm with an extra drizzle of lemon juice.

Nutritional Information (per serving):

Calories: 90 | Protein: 6g | Carbohydrates: 8g | Dietary Fiber: 4g | Sugars: 2g | Fat: 5g (Total), 1g (Saturated) | Cholesterol: 0mg | Sodium: 120mg

---

edamame & veggie salad

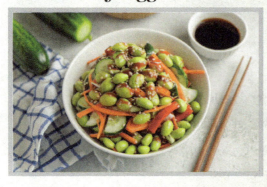

Ingredients (2 servings):

- ½ cup shelled edamame
- ½ cup diced cucumbers
- ¼ cup diced bell peppers
- ¼ cup shredded carrots
- 1 teaspoon sesame oil
- ½ teaspoon low-sodium soy sauce
- ¼ teaspoon black pepper

Instructions:

In a large bowl, combine edamame, cucumbers, bell peppers, and shredded carrots. - Drizzle with sesame oil and soy sauce. - Sprinkle with black pepper and toss well. - Serve chilled.

Nutritional Information (per serving):

Calories: 160 | Protein: 14g | Carbohydrates: 14g | Dietary Fiber: 5g | Sugars: 4g | Fat: 6g (Total), 1g (Saturated) | Cholesterol: 0mg | Sodium: 220mg

roasted brussels sprouts

Ingredients (2 servings):

- 2 cups Brussels sprouts, halved
- 1 teaspoon olive oil
- ½ teaspoon garlic powder
- ¼ teaspoon black pepper
- ¼ teaspoon salt
- 1 teaspoon balsamic vinegar

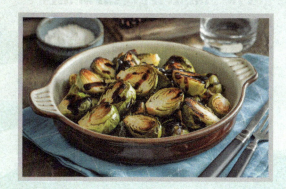

Instructions:

Preheat oven to 400°F (200°C). - In a bowl, toss Brussels sprouts with olive oil, garlic powder, black pepper, and salt. - Spread on a baking sheet lined with parchment paper. - Roast for 20-25 minutes, stirring halfway, until crispy and golden brown. - Drizzle with balsamic vinegar before serving.

Nutritional Information (per serving):

Calories: 150 | Protein: 8g | Carbohydrates: 18g | Dietary Fiber: 6g | Sugars: 5g | Fat: 6g (Total), 1g (Saturated) | Cholesterol: 0mg | Sodium: 200mg

---

high protein bean salad

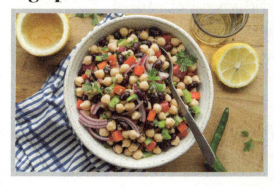

Ingredients (2 servings):

- ½ cup canned chickpeas, drained and rinsed
- ½ cup canned black beans, drained and rinsed
- ¼ cup diced red onions
- ¼ cup diced bell peppers
- 1 teaspoon olive oil
- 1 teaspoon lemon juice
- ½ teaspoon cumin
- ¼ teaspoon black pepper
- ¼ teaspoon salt

Instructions:

In a large bowl, combine chickpeas, black beans, red onions, and bell peppers. - Drizzle with olive oil and lemon juice. - Sprinkle with cumin, black pepper, and salt. - Toss well and serve chilled.

Nutritional Information (per serving):

Calories: 220 | Protein: 16g | Carbohydrates: 28g | Dietary Fiber: 10g | Sugars: 4g | Fat: 6g (Total), 1g (Saturated) | Cholesterol: 0mg | Sodium: 240mg

garlic roasted green beans

Ingredients (2 servings):

- 2 cups green beans, trimmed
- 1 teaspoon olive oil
- 2 cloves garlic, minced
- ¼ teaspoon black pepper
- ¼ teaspoon salt

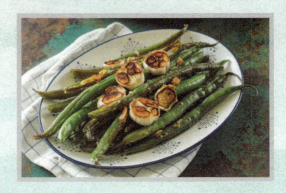

Instructions:

Preheat oven to 400°F (200°C). - In a bowl, toss green beans with olive oil, minced garlic, black pepper, and salt. - Spread on a baking sheet lined with parchment paper. - Roast for 12-15 minutes until tender-crisp. - Serve warm.

Nutritional Information (per serving):

Calories: 100 | Protein: 6g | Carbohydrates: 14g | Dietary Fiber: 5g | Sugars: 4g | Fat: 4g (Total), 0g (Saturated) | Cholesterol: 0mg | Sodium: 160mg

---

cucumber & chickpea salad

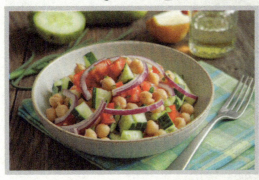

Ingredients (2 servings):

- ½ cup canned chickpeas, drained and rinsed
- ½ cup diced cucumbers
- ¼ cup diced tomatoes
- ¼ cup diced red onions
- 1 teaspoon olive oil
- 1 teaspoon apple cider vinegar
- ¼ teaspoon black pepper
- ¼ teaspoon salt

Instructions:

In a bowl, mix chickpeas, cucumbers, tomatoes, and red onions. - Drizzle with olive oil and apple cider vinegar. - Sprinkle with black pepper and salt. - Toss well and serve chilled.

Nutritional Information (per serving):

Calories: 180 | Protein: 14g | Carbohydrates: 22g | Dietary Fiber: 7g | Sugars: 5g | Fat: 5g (Total), 1g (Saturated) | Cholesterol: 0mg | Sodium: 180mg

baked sweet potato fries

Ingredients (2 servings):
- 1 medium sweet potato, peeled and cut into fries
- 1 teaspoon olive oil
- ½ teaspoon paprika
- ¼ teaspoon black pepper
- ¼ teaspoon salt

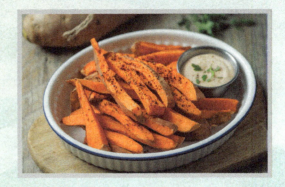

Instructions:

Preheat oven to 400°F (200°C). - In a bowl, toss sweet potato fries with olive oil, paprika, black pepper, and salt. - Spread evenly on a baking sheet lined with parchment paper. - Bake for 20-25 minutes, flipping halfway through, until crispy. - Serve warm.

Nutritional Information (per serving):

Calories: 220 | Protein: 4g | Carbohydrates: 38g | Dietary Fiber: 6g | Sugars: 8g | Fat: 6g (Total), 1g (Saturated) | Cholesterol: 0mg | Sodium: 140mg

---

creamy spinach & greek yogurt

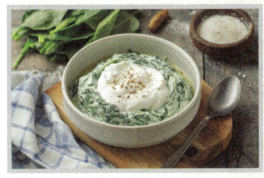

Ingredients (2 servings):
- 2 cups fresh spinach, chopped
- ½ cup Greek yogurt (plain, non-fat)
- 1 teaspoon olive oil
- 1 clove garlic, minced
- ¼ teaspoon black pepper
- ¼ teaspoon salt

Instructions:

Heat olive oil in a skillet over medium heat. - Add garlic and sauté for 1 minute until fragrant. - Stir in chopped spinach and cook for 2-3 minutes until wilted. - Remove from heat and mix in Greek yogurt, black pepper, and salt. - Serve warm.

Nutritional Information (per serving):

Calories: 110 | Protein: 10g | Carbohydrates: 7g | Dietary Fiber: 2g | Sugars: 3g | Fat: 4g (Total), 1g (Saturated) | Cholesterol: 5mg | Sodium: 180mg

veggie & lentil medley

Ingredients (2 servings):

- ½ cup cooked lentils
- ½ cup diced carrots
- ½ cup diced zucchini
- ¼ cup diced onions
- 1 teaspoon olive oil
- ½ teaspoon cumin
- ¼ teaspoon black pepper - ¼ teaspoon salt

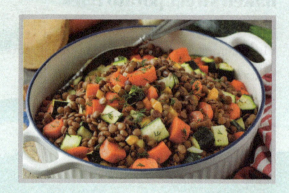

Instructions:

Heat olive oil in a skillet over medium heat. - Add onions, carrots, and zucchini, sauté for 3 minutes. - Stir in cooked lentils, cumin, black pepper, and salt. - Cook for another 2 minutes, stirring occasionally. - Serve warm.

Nutritional Information (per serving):

Calories: 180 | Protein: 12g | Carbohydrates: 28g | Dietary Fiber: 9g | Sugars: 5g | Fat: 4g (Total), 1g (Saturated) | Cholesterol: 0mg | Sodium: 190mg

---

roasted veggie mix

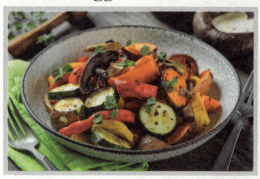

Ingredients (2 servings):

- ½ cup diced zucchini
- ½ cup diced bell peppers
- ½ cup diced sweet potatoes
- ½ cup diced mushrooms
- 1 teaspoon olive oil
- ½ teaspoon dried oregano
- ¼ teaspoon black pepper - ¼ teaspoon salt

Instructions:

Preheat oven to 400°F (200°C). - In a large bowl, toss all vegetables with olive oil, oregano, black pepper, and salt. - Spread evenly on a baking sheet lined with parchment paper. - Roast for 20-25 minutes, stirring halfway, until tender and slightly crispy. - Serve warm.

Nutritional Information (per serving):

Calories: 200 | Protein: 8g | Carbohydrates: 35g | Dietary Fiber: 8g | Sugars: 7g | Fat: 6g (Total), 1g (Saturated) | Cholesterol: 0mg | Sodium: 160mg

tomato and basil quinoa

Ingredients (2 servings):

- ½ cup dry quinoa
- 1 cup water
- ½ cup diced cherry tomatoes
- ¼ cup chopped fresh basil
- 1 teaspoon olive oil
- ¼ teaspoon black pepper
- ¼ teaspoon salt

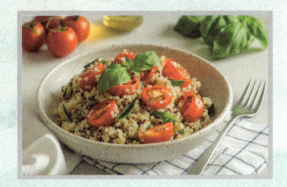

Instructions:

Rinse quinoa under cold water. - In a saucepan, bring quinoa and water to a boil. Reduce heat, cover, and simmer for 12-15 minutes until quinoa is tender. - Stir in diced cherry tomatoes, fresh basil, olive oil, black pepper, and salt. - Serve warm or chilled.

Nutritional Information (per serving):

Calories: 190 | Protein: 8g | Carbohydrates: 32g | Dietary Fiber: 5g | Sugars: 4g | Fat: 5g (Total), 1g (Saturated) | Cholesterol: 0mg | Sodium: 140mg

---

protein-rich coleslaw

Ingredients (2 servings):

- 1 cup shredded cabbage
- ½ cup shredded carrots
- ¼ cup Greek yogurt (plain, non-fat)
- 1 teaspoon apple cider vinegar
- ½ teaspoon Dijon mustard
- ¼ teaspoon black pepper
- ¼ teaspoon salt

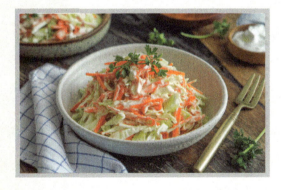

Instructions:

In a large bowl, mix shredded cabbage and carrots. - In a separate small bowl, whisk together Greek yogurt, apple cider vinegar, Dijon mustard, black pepper, and salt. - Pour dressing over the cabbage mixture and toss to coat. - Serve chilled.

Nutritional Information (per serving):

Calories: 120 | Protein: 10g | Carbohydrates: 12g | Dietary Fiber: 4g | Sugars: 6g | Fat: 3g (Total), 0g (Saturated) | Cholesterol: 5mg | Sodium: 180mg

snack recipes

Quick, Protein-Rich Snacks to Curb Cravings

Snacks can be a powerful tool to keep energy levels up and cravings at bay, especially when packed with protein. These quick and easy recipes provide a satisfying balance of nutrients to fuel your body between meals, whether you're at home, at work, or on the go.

protein energy balls

Ingredients (2 servings, 6 balls total):

- ½ cup rolled oats
- ¼ cup peanut butter
- 1 tablespoon honey
- 1 tablespoon chia seeds
- 1 scoop vanilla protein powder
- ¼ teaspoon cinnamon

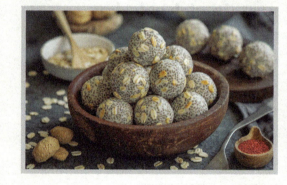

Instructions:

In a bowl, mix all ingredients until well combined. - Roll mixture into small balls (about 1 inch in diameter). - Place in the refrigerator for 30 minutes to firm up. - Store in an airtight container and enjoy as needed.

Nutritional Information (per serving - 3 balls):

Calories: 250 | Protein: 15g | Carbohydrates: 24g | Dietary Fiber: 5g | Sugars: 6g | Fat: 10g (Total), 2g (Saturated) | Cholesterol: 0mg | Sodium: 120mg

greek yogurt & berry bowl

Ingredients (2 servings):
- 1 cup Greek yogurt (plain, non-fat)
- ½ cup mixed berries (strawberries, blueberries, raspberries)
- 1 tablespoon honey
- 1 tablespoon chopped almonds

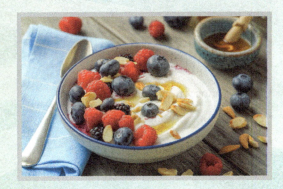

Instructions:

Divide Greek yogurt into two bowls. - Top with mixed berries, drizzle with honey, and sprinkle with chopped almonds. - Serve immediately.

Nutritional Information (per serving):

Calories: 220 | Protein: 18g | Carbohydrates: 24g | Dietary Fiber: 5g | Sugars: 12g | Fat: 5g (Total), 1g (Saturated) | Cholesterol: 5mg | Sodium: 75mg

---

cottage cheese & pineapple

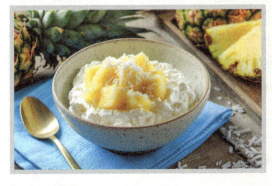

Ingredients (2 servings):
- 1 cup cottage cheese (low-fat)
- ½ cup diced pineapple
- 1 tablespoon shredded coconut (optional)

Instructions:

Divide cottage cheese into two bowls. - Top with diced pineapple and sprinkle with shredded coconut if desired. - Serve immediately.

Nutritional Information (per serving):

Calories: 180 | Protein: 20g | Carbohydrates: 15g | Dietary Fiber: 2g | Sugars: 10g | Fat: 4g (Total), 2g (Saturated) | Cholesterol: 10mg | Sodium: 320mg

peanut butter protein bars

Ingredients (2 servings, makes 4 bars):

- ½ cup rolled oats
- ¼ cup peanut butter
- 1 scoop chocolate protein powder
- 2 tablespoons almond milk
- 1 tablespoon honey

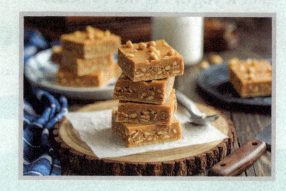

Instructions:

In a bowl, mix all ingredients until well combined. - Press the mixture into a small baking dish lined with parchment paper. - Refrigerate for at least 1 hour. - Slice into bars and serve.

Nutritional Information (per serving - 2 bars):

Calories: 280 | Protein: 22g | Carbohydrates: 28g | Dietary Fiber: 6g | Sugars: 8g | Fat: 10g (Total), 2g (Saturated) | Cholesterol: 0mg | Sodium: 150mg

―――

tuna & cucumber bites

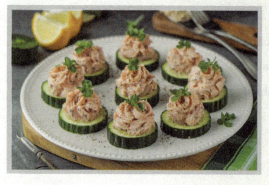

Ingredients (2 servings):

- ½ cup canned tuna, drained
- ½ teaspoon Dijon mustard
- ¼ teaspoon black pepper
- ¼ teaspoon salt
- 1 teaspoon Greek yogurt (plain)
- ½ cucumber, sliced into rounds

Instructions:

In a bowl, mix tuna, Dijon mustard, black pepper, salt, and Greek yogurt. - Place a small scoop of the tuna mixture onto each cucumber slice. - Serve immediately.

Nutritional Information (per serving - 6 bites):

Calories: 160 | Protein: 22g | Carbohydrates: 6g | Dietary Fiber: 2g | Sugars: 2g | Fat: 5g (Total), 1g (Saturated) | Cholesterol: 35mg | Sodium: 250mg

protein-packed trail mix

Ingredients (2 servings):
- ¼ cup almonds
- ¼ cup walnuts
- ¼ cup pumpkin seeds
- ¼ cup dried cranberries (unsweetened)
- ¼ cup dark chocolate chips (70% cacao or higher)

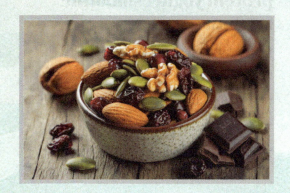

Instructions:

Mix all ingredients in a bowl. - Divide into two servings and store in an airtight container. - Enjoy as a protein-packed snack on the go.

Nutritional Information (per serving):

Calories: 320 | Protein: 14g | Carbohydrates: 24g | Dietary Fiber: 6g | Sugars: 10g | Fat: 22g (Total), 4g (Saturated) | Cholesterol: 0mg | Sodium: 10mg

---

avocado egg salad bites

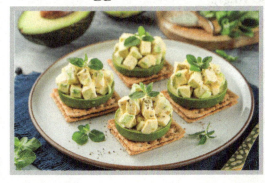

Ingredients (2 servings):
- 2 hard-boiled eggs, chopped
- ½ avocado, mashed
- ¼ teaspoon black pepper
- ¼ teaspoon salt
- 4 whole-grain crackers

Instructions:

In a bowl, mix chopped eggs, mashed avocado, black pepper, and salt. - Spoon mixture onto whole-grain crackers. - Serve immediately.

Nutritional Information (per serving - 2 bites):

Calories: 190 | Protein: 15g | Carbohydrates: 10g | Dietary Fiber: 4g | Sugars: 2g | Fat: 12g (Total), 3g (Saturated) | Cholesterol: 185mg | Sodium: 230mg

protein yogurt smoothie

Ingredients (2 servings):

- 1 cup Greek yogurt (plain, non-fat)
- ½ banana
- ½ cup mixed berries (strawberries, blueberries, raspberries)
- 1 scoop vanilla protein powder
- ½ cup almond milk (unsweetened)

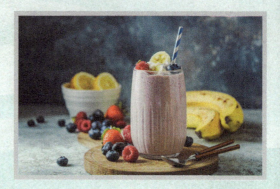

Instructions:

In a blender, combine all ingredients. - Blend until smooth. - Pour into glasses and serve immediately.

Nutritional Information (per serving):

Calories: 260 | Protein: 30g | Carbohydrates: 28g | Dietary Fiber: 6g | Sugars: 12g | Fat: 5g (Total), 1g (Saturated) | Cholesterol: 10mg | Sodium: 120mg

---

roasted chickpeas

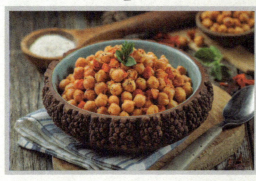

Ingredients (2 servings):

- 1 cup canned chickpeas, drained and rinsed
- 1 teaspoon olive oil
- ½ teaspoon paprika
- ¼ teaspoon black pepper
- ¼ teaspoon salt

Instructions:

Preheat oven to 400°F (200°C). - In a bowl, toss chickpeas with olive oil, paprika, black pepper, and salt. - Spread evenly on a baking sheet lined with parchment paper. - Roast for 25-30 minutes, stirring halfway, until crispy. - Let cool before serving.

Nutritional Information (per serving):

Calories: 180 | Protein: 12g | Carbohydrates: 26g | Dietary Fiber: 6g | Sugars: 3g | Fat: 5g (Total), 1g (Saturated) | Cholesterol: 0mg | Sodium: 200mg

almond butter & apple slices

Ingredients (2 servings):
- 1 medium apple, sliced
- 2 tablespoons almond butter

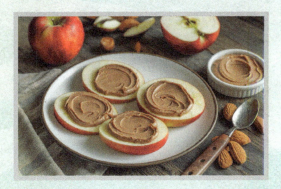

Instructions:

Slice the apple into wedges. - Spread almond butter on each slice. - Serve immediately.

Nutritional Information (per serving):

Calories: 210 | Protein: 8g | Carbohydrates: 28g | Dietary Fiber: 5g | Sugars: 18g | Fat: 10g (Total), 1g (Saturated) | Cholesterol: 0mg | Sodium: 5mg

---

turkey & cheese roll-ups

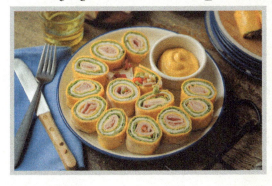

Ingredients (2 servings):
- 4 slices lean turkey breast
- 2 slices low-fat cheddar cheese
- 1 teaspoon Dijon mustard
- 4 small whole-wheat tortillas

Instructions:

Spread a thin layer of Dijon mustard on each tortilla. - Place one slice of turkey and half a slice of cheese on each tortilla. - Roll tightly and slice into bite-sized pieces if desired. - Serve immediately.

Nutritional Information (per serving - 2 roll-ups):

Calories: 220 | Protein: 26g | Carbohydrates: 18g | Dietary Fiber: 4g | Sugars: 2g | Fat: 6g (Total), 2g (Saturated) | Cholesterol: 40mg | Sodium: 360mg

protein veggie muffins

Ingredients (2 servings, makes 4 muffins):

- ½ cup egg whites
- ¼ cup grated zucchini
- ¼ cup diced bell peppers
- ¼ cup shredded low-fat cheddar cheese
- ¼ teaspoon garlic powder
- ¼ teaspoon black pepper
- ¼ teaspoon salt

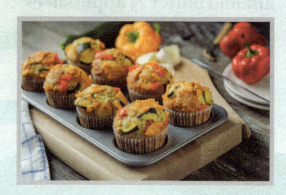

Instructions:

Preheat oven to 375°F (190°C). - In a bowl, whisk egg whites with garlic powder, black pepper, and salt. - Stir in grated zucchini, bell peppers, and cheddar cheese. - Pour mixture into a greased muffin tin, filling halfway. - Bake for 15-20 minutes until firm. - Let cool before serving.

Nutritional Information (per serving - 2 muffins):

Calories: 160 | Protein: 18g | Carbohydrates: 6g | Dietary Fiber: 2g | Sugars: 2g | Fat: 6g (Total), 2g (Saturated) | Cholesterol: 10mg | Sodium: 210mg

---

edamame snack bowl

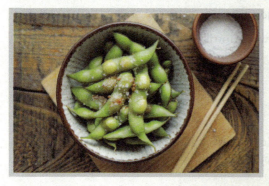

Ingredients (2 servings):

- 1 cup shelled edamame
- ½ teaspoon olive oil
- ¼ teaspoon sea salt
- ¼ teaspoon black pepper

Instructions:

Heat a skillet over medium heat. - Add edamame and olive oil, sauté for 2-3 minutes. - Sprinkle with sea salt and black pepper. - Serve warm or chilled.

Nutritional Information (per serving):

Calories: 180 | Protein: 16g | Carbohydrates: 14g | Dietary Fiber: 6g | Sugars: 2g | Fat: 7g (Total), 1g (Saturated) | Cholesterol: 0mg | Sodium: 160mg

egg salad celery boats

Ingredients (2 servings):
- 2 hard-boiled eggs, chopped
- 1 teaspoon Greek yogurt (plain, non-fat)
- ¼ teaspoon Dijon mustard
- ¼ teaspoon black pepper
- ¼ teaspoon salt
- 4 celery stalks, cut in half

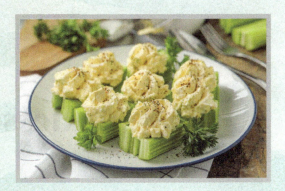

Instructions:

In a bowl, mix chopped eggs, Greek yogurt, Dijon mustard, black pepper, and salt. - Spoon mixture into celery stalks. - Serve immediately.

Nutritional Information (per serving - 4 boats):

Calories: 160 | Protein: 15g | Carbohydrates: 4g | Dietary Fiber: 2g | Sugars: 2g | Fat: 9g (Total), 3g (Saturated) | Cholesterol: 190mg | Sodium: 240mg

---

protein chocolate shake

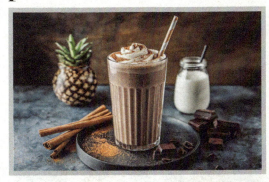

Ingredients (2 servings):
- 1 cup almond milk (unsweetened)
- 1 scoop chocolate protein powder
- ½ banana
- 1 tablespoon peanut butter
- ½ teaspoon cinnamon

Instructions:

In a blender, combine all ingredients. - Blend until smooth. - Pour into glasses and serve immediately.

Nutritional Information (per serving):

Calories: 260 | Protein: 28g | Carbohydrates: 22g | Dietary Fiber: 5g | Sugars: 10g | Fat: 8g (Total), 2g (Saturated) | Cholesterol: 10mg | Sodium: 140mg

dessert recipes

...

Guilt-Free Indulgences to Satisfy Your Sweet Tooth

Who says you can't enjoy dessert while maintaining a high-protein diet? These delicious treats are designed to satisfy your cravings without the guilt. Packed with protein and balanced with healthy ingredients, these recipes let you indulge while staying on track with your weight loss and fitness goals.

protein chocolate mousse

Ingredients (2 servings):

- 1 scoop chocolate protein powder
- ½ cup Greek yogurt (plain, non-fat)
- ½ cup unsweetened almond milk
- 1 tablespoon cocoa powder
- 1 teaspoon honey or stevia
- ½ teaspoon vanilla extract

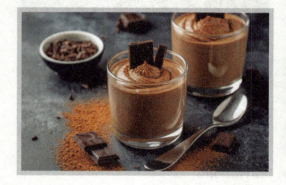

Instructions:

In a mixing bowl, whisk together protein powder, Greek yogurt, and almond milk until smooth. - Add cocoa powder, honey (or stevia), and vanilla extract, then mix until fluffy. - Chill for at least 30 minutes before serving.

Nutritional Information (per serving):

Calories: 180 | Protein: 22g | Carbohydrates: 10g | Dietary Fiber: 3g | Sugars: 5g | Fat: 5g (Total), 1g (Saturated) | Cholesterol: 10mg | Sodium: 180mg

greek yogurt cheesecake cups

Ingredients (2 servings):
- 1 cup Greek yogurt (plain, non-fat)
- ¼ cup low-fat cream cheese
- 1 tablespoon honey or maple syrup
- ½ teaspoon vanilla extract
- ¼ cup crushed whole-wheat graham crackers
- ¼ cup mixed berries (strawberries, blueberries, raspberries)

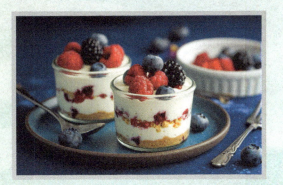

Instructions:

In a bowl, mix Greek yogurt, cream cheese, honey, and vanilla extract until smooth. - Divide the crushed graham crackers between two serving cups. - Spoon the yogurt mixture on top. - Top with mixed berries and chill for 15 minutes before serving.

Nutritional Information (per serving):

Calories: 210 | Protein: 18g | Carbohydrates: 22g | Dietary Fiber: 4g | Sugars: 12g | Fat: 6g (Total), 2g (Saturated) | Cholesterol: 10mg | Sodium: 140mg

---

high protein banana bread

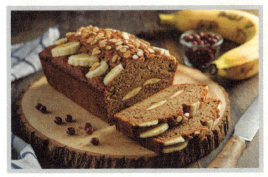

Ingredients (2 servings, makes 4 slices):
- ½ cup mashed ripe banana
- 1 scoop vanilla protein powder
- ¼ cup oat flour
- ¼ teaspoon baking soda
- ¼ teaspoon cinnamon
- 1 egg
- 1 tablespoon almond milk

Instructions:

Preheat oven to 350°F (175°C). - In a bowl, mix mashed banana, protein powder, oat flour, baking soda, and cinnamon. - Stir in egg and almond milk until well combined. - Pour into a small loaf pan and bake for 25-30 minutes. - Let cool before slicing.

Nutritional Information (per serving - 2 slices):

Calories: 220 | Protein: 20g | Carbohydrates: 28g | Dietary Fiber: 5g | Sugars: 10g | Fat: 5g (Total), 1g (Saturated) | Cholesterol: 55mg | Sodium: 200mg

chocolate avocado protein brownies

Ingredients (2 servings, makes 4 brownies):

- ½ cup mashed ripe avocado
- 1 scoop chocolate protein powder
- ¼ cup cocoa powder
- ¼ teaspoon baking powder
- ¼ teaspoon vanilla extract
- 1 tablespoon honey or maple syrup
- 1 egg

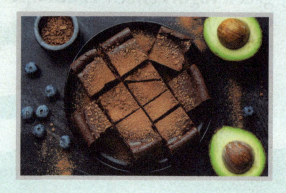

Instructions:

Preheat oven to 350°F (175°C). - In a bowl, mix mashed avocado, protein powder, cocoa powder, baking powder, vanilla extract, honey, and egg. - Stir until smooth. - Pour into a greased baking dish and bake for 20 minutes. - Let cool before slicing into brownies.

Nutritional Information (per serving - 2 brownies):

Calories: 250 | Protein: 22g | Carbohydrates: 18g | Dietary Fiber: 6g | Sugars: 7g | Fat: 10g (Total), 2g (Saturated) | Cholesterol: 60mg | Sodium: 180mg

---

vanilla protein pudding

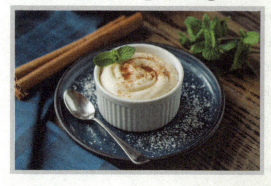

Ingredients (2 servings):

- 1 scoop vanilla protein powder
- 1 cup unsweetened almond milk
- 1 tablespoon chia seeds
- ½ teaspoon vanilla extract
- 1 teaspoon honey or stevia

Instructions:

In a mixing bowl, whisk together protein powder, almond milk, chia seeds, vanilla extract, and honey (or stevia). - Cover and refrigerate for at least 2 hours, stirring occasionally, until thickened. - Serve chilled.

Nutritional Information (per serving):

Calories: 180 | Protein: 20g | Carbohydrates: 12g | Dietary Fiber: 5g | Sugars: 5g | Fat: 6g (Total), 1g (Saturated) | Cholesterol: 0mg | Sodium: 120mg

peanut butter protein cookies

Ingredients (2 servings, makes 4 cookies):

- ½ cup natural peanut butter
- 1 scoop vanilla protein powder
- ¼ cup almond flour
- 1 tablespoon honey or stevia
- ¼ teaspoon baking soda
- 1 egg

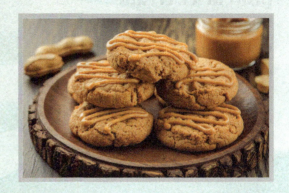

Instructions:

Preheat oven to 350°F (175°C). - In a bowl, mix peanut butter, protein powder, almond flour, honey, baking soda, and egg until a thick dough forms. - Divide into 4 small balls and flatten into cookie shapes. - Place on a parchment-lined baking sheet. - Bake for 10-12 minutes. - Let cool before serving.

Nutritional Information (per serving - 2 cookies):

Calories: 260 | Protein: 20g | Carbohydrates: 14g | Dietary Fiber: 4g | Sugars: 6g | Fat: 16g (Total), 4g (Saturated) | Cholesterol: 40mg | Sodium: 140mg

---

protein fruit crumble

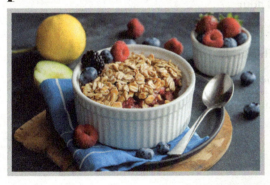

Ingredients (2 servings):

- 1 cup mixed berries (strawberries, blueberries, raspberries)
- 1 scoop vanilla protein powder
- ¼ cup rolled oats
- ¼ cup almond flour
- 1 tablespoon honey or maple syrup
- 1 teaspoon coconut oil

Instructions:

Preheat oven to 375°F (190°C). - In a small baking dish, layer mixed berries. - In a separate bowl, mix protein powder, oats, almond flour, honey, and coconut oil until crumbly. - Sprinkle over berries. - Bake for 15-20 minutes until golden brown. - Serve warm.

Nutritional Information (per serving):

Calories: 220 | Protein: 18g | Carbohydrates: 28g | Dietary Fiber: 6g | Sugars: 10g | Fat: 6g (Total), 1g (Saturated) | Cholesterol: 0mg | Sodium: 120mg

protein ice cream

Ingredients (2 servings):

- 1 frozen banana
- 1 scoop vanilla protein powder
- ½ cup unsweetened almond milk
- ½ teaspoon vanilla extract

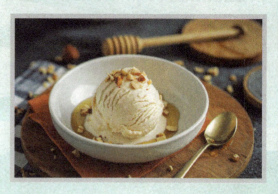

Instructions:

In a blender, combine all ingredients. - Blend until smooth and creamy. - Transfer to a container and freeze for 1-2 hours until firm. - Serve chilled.

Nutritional Information (per serving):

Calories: 200 | Protein: 22g | Carbohydrates: 24g | Dietary Fiber: 5g | Sugars: 12g | Fat: 3g (Total), 0g (Saturated) | Cholesterol: 0mg | Sodium: 100mg

---

chia seed protein cookies

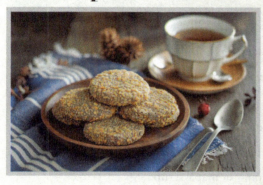

Ingredients (2 servings, makes 4 cookies):

- ½ cup almond flour
- 1 scoop vanilla protein powder
- 1 tablespoon chia seeds
- 1 tablespoon honey or stevia
- ¼ teaspoon cinnamon
- 1 egg

Instructions:

Preheat oven to 350°F (175°C). - In a bowl, mix almond flour, protein powder, chia seeds, honey, cinnamon, and egg until dough forms. - Shape into 4 small cookies and place on a baking sheet. - Bake for 10-12 minutes. - Let cool before serving.

Nutritional Information (per serving - 2 cookies):

Calories: 210 | Protein: 18g | Carbohydrates: 14g | Dietary Fiber: 5g | Sugars: 6g | Fat: 10g (Total), 2g (Saturated) | Cholesterol: 35mg | Sodium: 110mg

protein cheesecake bites

Ingredients (2 servings, makes 4 bites):

- ½ cup Greek yogurt (plain, non-fat)
- ¼ cup low-fat cream cheese
- 1 scoop vanilla protein powder
- 1 tablespoon honey or stevia
- ¼ cup crushed whole-wheat graham crackers

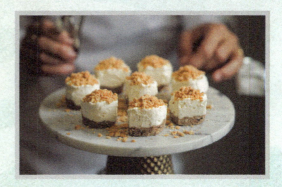

Instructions:

In a bowl, mix Greek yogurt, cream cheese, protein powder, and honey until smooth. - Spoon mixture into a silicone mold or small paper cups. - Sprinkle crushed graham crackers on top. - Freeze for at least 1 hour before serving.

Nutritional Information (per serving - 2 bites):

Calories: 180 | Protein: 20g | Carbohydrates: 18g | Dietary Fiber: 3g | Sugars: 8g | Fat: 5g (Total), 2g (Saturated) | Cholesterol: 15mg | Sodium: 120mg

---

chocolate protein pancake stack

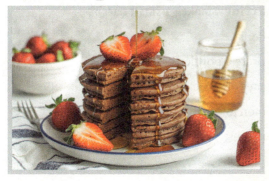

Ingredients (2 servings, makes 6 small pancakes):

- 1 scoop chocolate protein powder
- ½ cup oat flour
- 1 teaspoon cocoa powder
- ½ teaspoon baking powder
- 1 egg
- ½ cup unsweetened almond milk
- 1 teaspoon honey or stevia

Instructions:

In a bowl, mix protein powder, oat flour, cocoa powder, and baking powder. - Add egg, almond milk, and honey, then whisk until smooth. - Heat a non-stick skillet over medium heat. - Pour small amounts of batter to form pancakes. - Cook for 2 minutes on one side, then flip and cook for another 1-2 minutes. - Stack pancakes and serve with fresh berries or a drizzle of honey.

Nutritional Information (per serving - 3 pancakes):

Calories: 260 | Protein: 26g | Carbohydrates: 28g | Dietary Fiber: 6g | Sugars: 5g | Fat: 6g (Total), 1g (Saturated) | Cholesterol: 55mg | Sodium: 220mg

strawberry protein sorbet

Ingredients (2 servings):

- 1 cup frozen strawberries
- 1 scoop vanilla protein powder
- ½ cup unsweetened almond milk
- ½ teaspoon vanilla extract

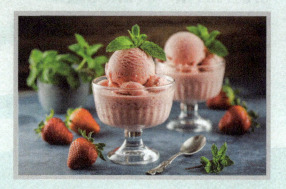

Instructions:

In a blender, combine all ingredients. - Blend until smooth and thick. - Serve immediately or freeze for 30 minutes for a firmer texture.

Nutritional Information (per serving):

Calories: 180 | Protein: 22g | Carbohydrates: 20g | Dietary Fiber: 4g | Sugars: 10g | Fat: 2g (Total), 0g (Saturated) | Cholesterol: 0mg | Sodium: 100mg

---

protein lemon bars

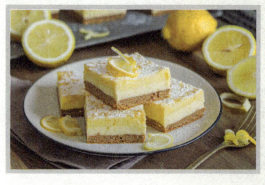

Ingredients (2 servings, makes 4 small bars):

- ½ cup almond flour
- 1 scoop vanilla protein powder
- 1 tablespoon honey or stevia
- 1 tablespoon lemon juice
- ½ teaspoon lemon zest
- 1 egg

Instructions:

Preheat oven to 350°F (175°C). - In a bowl, mix almond flour, protein powder, honey, lemon juice, lemon zest, and egg. - Pour mixture into a small baking dish. - Bake for 15-20 minutes. - Let cool before slicing into bars.

Nutritional Information (per serving - 2 bars):

Calories: 220 | Protein: 18g | Carbohydrates: 16g | Dietary Fiber: 4g | Sugars: 6g | Fat: 8g (Total), 2g (Saturated) | Cholesterol: 55mg | Sodium: 140mg

banana chocolate chip protein muffins

Ingredients (2 servings, makes 4 muffins):

- ½ cup mashed banana
- 1 scoop chocolate protein powder
- ¼ cup oat flour
- ¼ teaspoon baking powder
- 1 tablespoon dark chocolate chips
- 1 egg

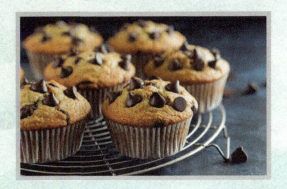

Instructions:

Preheat oven to 350°F (175°C). - In a bowl, mix mashed banana, protein powder, oat flour, baking powder, and egg. - Stir in dark chocolate chips. - Pour into a greased muffin tin. - Bake for 18-20 minutes. - Let cool before serving.

Nutritional Information (per serving - 2 muffins):

Calories: 240 | Protein: 22g | Carbohydrates: 28g | Dietary Fiber: 5g | Sugars: 10g | Fat: 6g (Total), 2g (Saturated) | Cholesterol: 50mg | Sodium: 160mg

---

coconut protein truffles

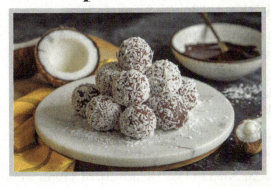

Ingredients (2 servings, makes 6 truffles):

- ½ cup shredded coconut (unsweetened)
- 1 scoop vanilla protein powder
- 1 tablespoon coconut oil
- 1 tablespoon honey or stevia
- ½ teaspoon vanilla extract

Instructions:

In a bowl, mix shredded coconut, protein powder, coconut oil, honey, and vanilla extract. - Roll into small balls. - Place in the refrigerator for at least 30 minutes before serving.

Nutritional Information (per serving - 3 truffles):

Calories: 220 | Protein: 18g | Carbohydrates: 14g | Dietary Fiber: 4g | Sugars: 6g | Fat: 12g (Total), 4g (Saturated) | Cholesterol: 0mg | Sodium: 80mg

60 day meal plan

...

DAY 1: Breakfast: Protein-Packed Omelette (p.1) - Lunch: Grilled Chicken Salad (p.12) - Dinner: Garlic Herb Grilled Salmon (p.28) - Snack 1: Protein Energy Balls (p.60) - Snack 2: Roasted Chickpeas (p.65)

DAY 2: Breakfast: Greek Yogurt Parfait (p.2) - Lunch: Tuna Avocado Wrap (p.13) - Dinner: Chicken and Broccoli Stir-fry (p.29) - Snack 1: Almond Butter & Apple Slices (p.65) - Snack 2: Cottage Cheese & Pineapple (p.62)

DAY 3: Breakfast: Spinach and Egg Muffins (p.2) - Lunch: Quinoa and Chickpea Bowl (p.13) - Dinner: High-Protein Beef Stir-fry (p.31) - Snack 1: Greek Yogurt & Berry Bowl (p.61) - Snack 2: Roasted Brussels Sprouts (p.55)

DAY 4: Breakfast: High Protein Pancakes (p.3) - Lunch: High Protein Cobb Salad (p.14) - Dinner: Zucchini Noodles with Turkey Meatballs (p.34) - Snack 1: Tuna & Cucumber Bites (p.63) - Snack 2: Egg Salad Celery Boats (p.67) - Dessert: Chocolate Protein Pancake Stack (p.73)

DAY 5: Breakfast: Breakfast Burrito (p.3) - Lunch: Turkey and Veggie Sandwich (p.14) - Dinner: Herb Roasted Chicken Breast (p.36) - Snack 1: Avocado Egg Salad Bites (p.63) - Snack 2: Edamame Snack Bowl (p.66)

DAY 6: Breakfast: Cottage Cheese and Fruit Bowl (p.4) - Lunch: Lentil Soup (p.15) - Dinner: Shrimp and Vegetable Skewers (p.32) - Snack 1: Protein Yogurt Smoothie (p.64) - Snack 2: Baked Sweet Potato Fries (p.57)

DAY 7: Breakfast: Avocado and Egg Toast (p.4) - Lunch: Chicken Caesar Wrap (p.15) - Dinner: Baked Tilapia with Veggies (p.37) - Snack 1: Turkey & Cheese Roll-ups (p.65) - Snack 2: Cucumber & Chickpea Salad (p.56) - Dessert: Protein Ice Cream (p.72)

DAY 8: Breakfast: Chia Seed Protein Pudding (p.5) - Lunch: Greek Salad with Grilled Chicken (p.16) - Dinner: High-Protein Taco Salad (p.38) - Snack 1: Protein-Packed Trail Mix (p.63) - Snack 2: Roasted Garlic Green Beans (p.55) - Dessert: Peanut Butter Protein Cookies (p.71)

DAY 9: Breakfast: Smoked Salmon Bagel (p.5) - Lunch: Egg Salad Lettuce Wraps (p.16) - Dinner: Spaghetti Squash with Turkey Bolognese (p.38) - Snack 1: Cottage Cheese & Pineapple (p.62) - Snack 2: Tomato and Basil Quinoa (p.59)

DAY 10: Breakfast: Almond Butter Banana Toast (p.6) - Lunch: Salmon Sushi Bowl (p.17) - Dinner: Chicken Parmesan (Low-Carb) (p.39) - Snack 1: Egg and Tuna Salad (p.26) - Snack 2: Creamy Spinach & Greek Yogurt (p.57)

DAY 11: Breakfast: Breakfast Egg and Veggie Skillet (p.6) - Lunch: Black Bean Burrito Bowl (p.17) - Dinner: Grilled

HIGH PROTEIN COOKBOOK

Pork Chops with Veggies (p.40) - Snack 1: Greek Yogurt & Berry Bowl (p.61) - Snack 2: Veggie & Lentil Medley (p.58) - Dessert: Protein Cheesecake Bites (p.73)

DAY 12: Breakfast: Berry Smoothie Bowl (p.7) - Lunch: Chicken Fajita Salad (p.18) - Dinner: Teriyaki Chicken Protein Bowl (p.41) - Snack 1: Almond Butter & Apple Slices (p.65) - Snack 2: Roasted Chickpeas (p.65)

DAY 13: Breakfast: Turkey Sausage and Egg Muffins (p.7) - Lunch: Protein Pasta Primavera (p.18) - Dinner: Lemon Garlic Chicken Breasts (p.41) - Snack 1: Turkey & Cheese Roll-ups (p.65) - Snack 2: Roasted Veggie Mix (p.58)

DAY 14: Breakfast: Overnight Protein Oats (p.8) - Lunch: Shrimp and Quinoa Salad (p.19) - Dinner: Baked Salmon with Dill Sauce (p.42) - Snack 1: Avocado Egg Salad Bites (p.63) - Snack 2: Protein Yogurt Smoothie (p.64) - Dessert: Protein Lemon Bars (p.74)

DAY 15: Breakfast: Scrambled Egg Whites with Veggies (p.8) - Lunch: Avocado Chicken Wrap (p.19) - Dinner: Turkey Zucchini Burgers (p.42) - Snack 1: Roasted Brussels Sprouts (p.55) - Snack 2: Cottage Cheese & Pineapple (p.62) - Dessert: Protein Chocolate Mousse (p.68)

DAY 16: Breakfast: Banana Nut Protein Bread (p.9) - Lunch: High Protein Chili (p.20) - Dinner: Protein Veggie Lasagna (p.43) - Snack 1: Protein-Packed Trail Mix (p.63) - Snack 2: Tomato and Basil Quinoa (p.59)

DAY 17: Breakfast: Quinoa Breakfast Bowl (p.9) - Lunch: Mediterranean Chicken Bowl (p.20) - Dinner: Chickpea & Quinoa Salad (p.44) - Snack 1: Roasted Chickpeas (p.65) - Snack 2: Greek Yogurt & Berry Bowl (p.61)

DAY 18: Breakfast: Egg and Cheese Wrap (p.10) - Lunch: Asian Tofu Salad (p.21) - Dinner: High-Protein Lentil Curry (p.45) - Snack 1: Edamame Snack Bowl (p.66) - Snack 2: Protein Veggie Muffins (p.66) - Dessert: Chia Seed Protein Cookies (p.72)

DAY 19: Breakfast: Tofu Scramble (p.10) - Lunch: Turkey Burger Lettuce Wrap (p.21) - Dinner: Black Bean Veggie Burger (p.45) - Snack 1: Turkey & Cheese Roll-ups (p.65) - Snack 2: Creamy Spinach & Greek Yogurt (p.57)

DAY 20: Breakfast: Protein French Toast (p.11) - Lunch: Lentil and Veggie Stir-fry (p.22) - Dinner: Mushroom & Lentil Tacos (p.48) - Snack 1: Roasted Garlic Green Beans (p.55) - Snack 2: Avocado Egg Salad Bites (p.63)

DAY 21: Breakfast: Protein-Packed Omelette (p.1) - Lunch: Salmon Avocado Salad (p.22) - Dinner: Vegetarian Eggplant Parmesan (p.50) - Snack 1: Greek Yogurt Cheesecake Cups (p.69) - Snack 2: Almond Butter & Apple Slices (p.65) - Dessert: Coconut Protein Truffles (p.75)

DAY 22: Breakfast: Greek Yogurt Parfait (p.2) - Lunch: Chickpea Protein Wrap (p.23) - Dinner: Vegan Buddha Bowl (p.47) - Snack 1: Roasted Veggie Mix (p.58) - Snack 2: Protein Yogurt Smoothie (p.64)

DAY 23: Breakfast: Spinach and Egg Muffins (p.2) - Lunch: Spinach & Turkey Meatballs (p.23) - Dinner: Tofu & Veggie Stir-fry (p.44) - Snack 1: Tuna & Cucumber Bites (p.63) - Snack 2: Egg Salad Celery Boats (p.67)

DAY 24: Breakfast: High Protein Pancakes (p.3) - Lunch: Spicy Tuna Salad Bowl (p.24) - Dinner: Chickpea Salad Sandwich (p.49) - Snack 1: Cucumber & Chickpea Salad (p.56) - Snack 2: Protein Chocolate Shake (p.67) - Dessert: Protein Fruit Crumble (p.71)

DAY 25: Breakfast: Breakfast Burrito (p.3) - Lunch: Veggie Omelette Wrap (p.24) - Dinner: Black Bean Enchiladas (p.50) - Snack 1: Roasted Brussels Sprouts (p.55) - Snack 2: Protein Energy Balls (p.60)

DAY 26: Breakfast: Cottage Cheese and Fruit Bowl (p.4) - Lunch: High Protein Buddha Bowl (p.25) - Dinner: Lentil and Mushroom Burgers (p.51) - Snack 1: Turkey & Cheese Roll-ups (p.65) - Snack 2: Tomato and Basil Quinoa (p.59)

DAY 27: Breakfast: Avocado and Egg Toast (p.4) - Lunch: Egg and Tuna Salad (p.26) - Dinner: Quinoa and Veggie Protein Bowl (p.51) - Snack 1: Edamame Snack Bowl (p.66) - Snack 2: Greek Yogurt & Berry Bowl (p.61) - Dessert: Strawberry Protein Sorbet (p.74)

DAY 28: Breakfast: Chia Seed Protein Pudding (p.5) - Lunch: Grilled Chicken and Veggie Wrap (p.26) - Dinner: High Protein Pasta with Spinach and Chickpeas (p.47) - Snack 1: Almond Butter & Apple Slices (p.65) - Snack 2: Roasted Chickpeas (p.65)

DAY 29: Breakfast: Smoked Salmon Bagel (p.5) - Lunch: Steak Salad with Protein Dressing (p.27) - Dinner: Herb Roasted Chicken Breast (p.36) - Snack 1: Roasted Garlic Green Beans (p.55) - Snack 2: Protein-Packed Trail Mix (p.63) - Dessert: Chocolate Protein Mousse (p.68)

DAY 30: Breakfast: Almond Butter Banana Toast (p.6) - Lunch: Protein-Packed Turkey Soup (p.27) - Dinner: Grilled Tuna Steaks (p.35) - Snack 1: Greek Yogurt Cheesecake Cups (p.69) - Snack 2: Cottage Cheese & Pineapple (p.62)

DAY 31: Breakfast: Breakfast Egg and Veggie Skillet (p.6) - Lunch: Grilled Chicken Salad (p.12) - Dinner: Spicy Shrimp Stir-fry (p.39) - Snack 1: Egg Salad Celery Boats (p.67) - Snack 2: Roasted Brussels Sprouts (p.55)

DAY 32: Breakfast: Berry Smoothie Bowl (p.7) - Lunch: Tuna Avocado Wrap (p.13) - Dinner: Spicy Bean Chili (p.46) - Snack 1: Turkey & Cheese Roll-ups (p.65) - Snack 2: Baked Sweet Potato Fries (p.57) - Dessert: Peanut Butter Protein Cookies (p.71)

DAY 33: Breakfast: Turkey Sausage and Egg Muffins (p.7) - Lunch: Quinoa and Chickpea Bowl (p.13) - Dinner: High-Protein Taco Salad (p.38) - Snack 1: Almond Butter & Apple Slices (p.65) - Snack 2: Roasted Chickpeas (p.65)

DAY 34: Breakfast: Overnight Protein Oats (p.8) - Lunch: High Protein Cobb Salad (p.14) - Dinner: Grilled Chicken with Avocado Salsa (p.33) - Snack 1: Edamame Snack Bowl (p.66) - Snack 2: Protein Yogurt Smoothie (p.64)

DAY 35: Breakfast: Scrambled Egg Whites with Veggies (p.8) - Lunch: Turkey and Veggie Sandwich (p.14) - Dinner: Zucchini Noodles with Turkey Meatballs (p.34) - Snack 1: Avocado Egg Salad Bites (p.63) - Snack 2: Protein Energy Balls (p.60) - Dessert: Chocolate Avocado Protein Brownies (p.69)

DAY 36: Breakfast: Banana Nut Protein Bread (p.9) - Lunch: Lentil Soup (p.15) - Dinner: Baked Salmon with Dill Sauce (p.42) - Snack 1: Roasted Brussels Sprouts (p.55) - Snack 2: Cucumber & Chickpea Salad (p.56)

DAY 37: Breakfast: Quinoa Breakfast Bowl (p.9) - Lunch: Chicken Caesar Wrap (p.15) - Dinner: Spaghetti Squash with Turkey Bolognese (p.38) - Snack 1: Cottage Cheese & Pineapple (p.62) - Snack 2: Tomato and Basil Quinoa (p.59)

DAY 38: Breakfast: Egg and Cheese Wrap (p.10) - Lunch: Greek Salad with Grilled Chicken (p.16) - Dinner: Vegetarian Eggplant Parmesan (p.50) - Snack 1: Almond Butter & Apple Slices (p.65) - Snack 2: Roasted Chickpeas (p.65) - Dessert: Protein Cheesecake Bites (p.73)

DAY 39: Breakfast: Tofu Scramble (p.10) - Lunch: Egg Salad Lettuce Wraps (p.16) - Dinner: Mushroom & Lentil Tacos (p.48) - Snack 1: Turkey & Cheese Roll-ups (p.65) - Snack 2: Protein Chocolate Shake (p.67)

DAY 40: Breakfast: Protein French Toast (p.11) - Lunch: Salmon Sushi Bowl (p.17) - Dinner: Grilled Pork Chops with Veggies (p.40) - Snack 1: Greek Yogurt & Berry Bowl (p.61) - Snack 2: Roasted Veggie Mix (p.58)

DAY 41: Breakfast: Protein-Packed Omelette (p.1) - Lunch: Chicken Fajita Salad (p.18) - Dinner: Chickpea & Quinoa Salad (p.44) - Snack 1: Edamame Snack Bowl (p.66) - Snack 2: Greek Yogurt Cheesecake Cups (p.69)

DAY 42: Breakfast: Greek Yogurt Parfait (p.2) - Lunch: Shrimp and Quinoa Salad (p.19) - Dinner: High-Protein Lentil Curry (p.45) - Snack 1: Egg Salad Celery Boats (p.67) - Snack 2: Protein Fruit Crumble (p.71)

DAY 43: Breakfast: Spinach and Egg Muffins (p.2) - Lunch: Avocado Chicken Wrap (p.19) - Dinner: High Protein Pasta with Spinach and Chickpeas (p.47) - Snack 1: Protein-Packed Trail Mix (p.63) - Snack 2: Roasted Garlic Green Beans (p.55) - Dessert: Protein Lemon Bars (p.74)

DAY 44: Breakfast: High Protein Pancakes (p.3) - Lunch: High Protein Chili (p.20) - Dinner: Black Bean Veggie Burger (p.45) - Snack 1: Tuna & Cucumber Bites (p.63) - Snack 2: Cottage Cheese & Pineapple (p.62)

DAY 45: Breakfast: Breakfast Burrito (p.3) - Lunch: Mediterranean Chicken Bowl (p.20) - Dinner: Vegan Buddha Bowl (p.47) - Snack 1: Protein Energy Balls (p.60) - Snack 2: Roasted Chickpeas (p.65)

DAY 46: Breakfast: Cottage Cheese and Fruit Bowl (p.4) - Lunch: Asian Tofu Salad (p.21) - Dinner: Chickpea Salad Sandwich (p.49) - Snack 1: Almond Butter & Apple Slices (p.65) - Snack 2: Roasted Brussels Sprouts (p.55) - Dessert: Protein Cheesecake Bites (p.73)

DAY 47: Breakfast: Avocado and Egg Toast (p.4) - Lunch: Turkey Burger Lettuce Wrap (p.21) - Dinner: Lentil and Mushroom Burgers (p.51) - Snack 1: Edamame Snack Bowl (p.66) - Snack 2: Greek Yogurt & Berry Bowl (p.61)

DAY 48: Breakfast: Chia Seed Protein Pudding (p.5) - Lunch: Lentil and Veggie Stir-fry (p.22) - Dinner: Vegetarian Eggplant Parmesan (p.50) - Snack 1: Egg Salad Celery Boats (p.67) - Snack 2: Protein Yogurt Smoothie (p.64)

DAY 49: Breakfast: Smoked Salmon Bagel (p.5) - Lunch: Salmon Avocado Salad (p.22) - Dinner: Quinoa and Veggie Protein Bowl (p.51) - Snack 1: Turkey & Cheese Roll-ups (p.65) - Snack 2: Tomato and Basil Quinoa (p.59) - Dessert: Protein Ice Cream (p.72)

DAY 50: Breakfast: Almond Butter Banana Toast (p.6) - Lunch: Chickpea Protein Wrap (p.23) - Dinner: Spaghetti Squash with Turkey Bolognese (p.38) - Snack 1: Roasted Veggie Mix (p.58) - Snack 2: Protein Chocolate Shake (p.67)

DAY 51: Breakfast: Breakfast Egg and Veggie Skillet (p.6) - Lunch: Spinach & Turkey Meatballs (p.23) - Dinner: Mushroom & Lentil Tacos (p.48) - Snack 1: Avocado Egg Salad Bites (p.63) - Snack 2: Baked Sweet Potato Fries (p.57)

DAY 52: Breakfast: Berry Smoothie Bowl (p.7) - Lunch: Spicy Tuna Salad Bowl (p.24) - Dinner: High-Protein Lentil Curry (p.45) - Snack 1: Greek Yogurt Cheesecake Cups (p.69) - Snack 2: Protein Fruit Crumble (p.71) - Dessert: Coconut Protein Truffles (p.75)

DAY 53: Breakfast: Turkey Sausage and Egg Muffins (p.7) - Lunch: Veggie Omelette Wrap (p.24) - Dinner: Black Bean Enchiladas (p.50) - Snack 1: Cottage Cheese & Pineapple (p.62) - Snack 2: Roasted Garlic Green Beans (p.55)

DAY 54: Breakfast: Overnight Protein Oats (p.8) - Lunch: High Protein Buddha Bowl (p.25) - Dinner: Baked Tilapia with Veggies (p.37) - Snack 1: Roasted Chickpeas (p.65) - Snack 2: Protein Energy Balls (p.60)

DAY 55: Breakfast: Scrambled Egg Whites with Veggies (p.8) - Lunch: Egg and Tuna Salad (p.26) - Dinner: Grilled Pork Chops with Veggies (p.40) - Snack 1: Almond Butter & Apple Slices (p.65) - Snack 2: Roasted Brussels Sprouts (p.55)

DAY 56: Breakfast: Banana Nut Protein Bread (p.9) - Lunch: Grilled Chicken and Veggie Wrap (p.26) - Dinner: Teriyaki Chicken Protein Bowl (p.41) - Snack 1: Protein Yogurt Smoothie (p.64) - Snack 2: Roasted Veggie Mix (p.58) - Dessert: Strawberry Protein Sorbet (p.74)

DAY 57: Breakfast: Quinoa Breakfast Bowl (p.9) - Lunch: Steak Salad with Protein Dressing (p.27) - Dinner: Baked Salmon with Dill Sauce (p.42) - Snack 1: Roasted Chickpeas (p.65) - Snack 2: Cucumber & Chickpea Salad (p.56)

DAY 58: Breakfast: Egg and Cheese Wrap (p.10) - Lunch: Protein-Packed Turkey Soup (p.27) - Dinner: High-Protein Taco Salad (p.38) - Snack 1: Edamame Snack Bowl (p.66) - Snack 2: Roasted Brussels Sprouts (p.55)

DAY 59: Breakfast: Tofu Scramble (p.10) - Lunch: Mediterranean Chicken Bowl (p.20) - Dinner: Vegetarian Eggplant Parmesan (p.50) - Snack 1: Protein Energy Balls (p.60) - Snack 2: Protein Chocolate Shake (p.67)

DAY 60: Breakfast: Protein French Toast (p.11) - Lunch: Lentil and Veggie Stir-fry (p.22) - Dinner: High Protein Pasta with Spinach and Chickpeas (p.47) - Snack 1: Greek Yogurt Cheesecake Cups (p.69) - Snack 2: Roasted Garlic Green Beans (p.55)

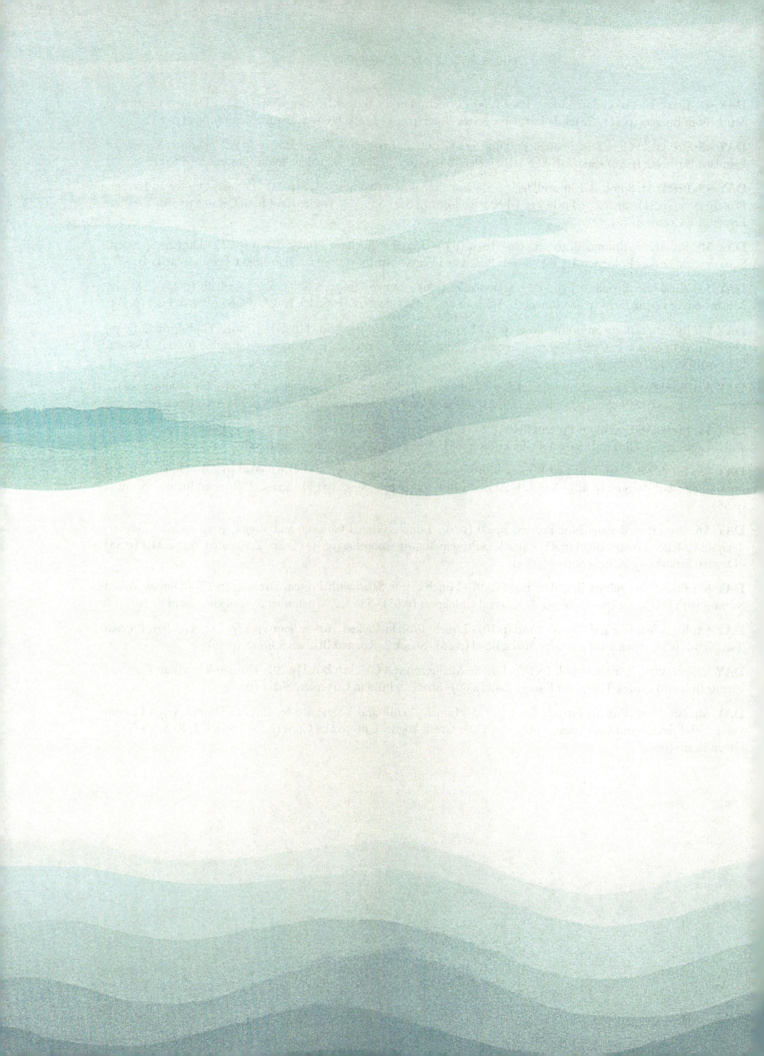

acknowledgments

I want to express my deepest gratitude to everyone who supported me in creating this cookbook. Writing a book is never a solo journey, and I am incredibly thankful for the encouragement, inspiration, and guidance I received along the way.

To my readers—thank you for trusting me to be a part of your health and fitness journey. Your dedication to a high-protein lifestyle motivates me to continue sharing recipes and insights that make clean eating both enjoyable and sustainable.

To my family and friends—your unwavering support, patience, and honest feedback have been invaluable throughout this process. I appreciate every meal we've shared, every recipe you've tested, and every word of encouragement you've given me.

A special thanks to my publishing team and everyone who helped shape this book into what it is today. Your expertise, commitment, and belief in my vision have made all the difference.

Finally, to those striving to improve their health through nutrition—this book is for you. I hope it serves as a practical guide and a source of inspiration as you fuel your body with wholesome, protein-rich meals.

Eat well, stay strong, and enjoy the journey!

— **Mark Primitive**

---

about the author

Mark Primitive is a dedicated nutrition enthusiast and cookbook author passionate about helping people transform their health through high-protein, whole-food eating. With a background in fitness and a deep understanding of how food fuels the body, Mark has spent years researching and developing easy, delicious, and nutritious recipes tailored for weight loss, muscle maintenance, and overall well-being.

He is also the author of **"ZERO-STRESS Carnivore Diet Cookbook"**, where he explores the benefits of a meat-based diet for optimal performance and fat loss. Through his work, Mark aims to make clean eating accessible to everyone, whether you're a fitness enthusiast, an athlete, or someone simply looking to improve your relationship with food.

When he's not writing or cooking, Mark enjoys weight training, hiking, and experimenting with new meal prep techniques to maximize nutrition and efficiency.

To stay updated with Mark's latest recipes and insights, follow him online and join his community of health-conscious individuals taking charge of their nutrition.